HEAL.

BY JOSEPHINE

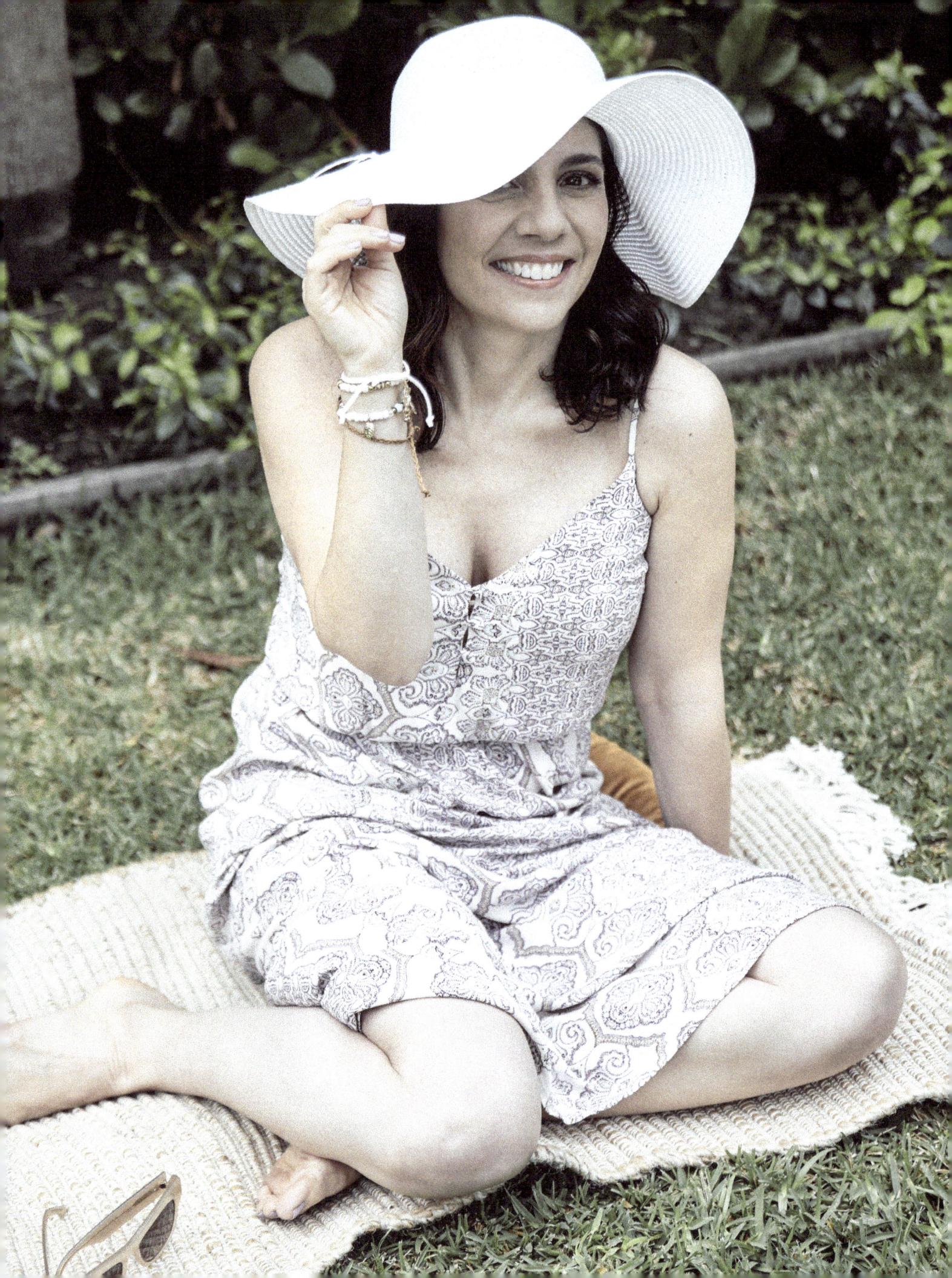

HEAL.

BY JOSEPHINE

Discover products,
homeopathic remedies,
and concepts to awaken
the mind, body and soul

JOSEPHINE ZAPPIA

First published in 2023 by Dean Publishing
PO Box 119
Mt. Macedon, Victoria, 3441
Australia
deanpublishing.com

DEAN PUBLISHING

Cataloguing-in-Publication Data
National Library of Australia
Title: HEAL. By Josephine
Edition: 1st edn
ISBN: 978-1-925452-63-1
Category: Holistic Medicine/Homeopathy/Healing

Photography: Yasmin Mund, www.yasminmund.com

The views and opinions expressed in this book are those of the author and do not necessarily reflect the official policy or position of any other agency, publisher, organisation, employer or company. Assumptions made in the analysis are not reflective of the position of any entity other than the author(s) — and, these views are always subject to change, revision, and rethinking at any time. The author, publisher or organisations are not to be held responsible for misuse, reuse, recycled and cited and/or uncited copies of content within this book by others.

This book and its natural remedies act as a personal guide only and are not to be used without appropriate consultation with your doctor. This book is not intended as a substitute for the medical advice of physicians. The reader should regularly consult a physician in matters relating to his/her health and particularly with respect to any symptoms that may require diagnosis or medical attention. The ideas within this book are only the opinion of the author and are not intended to replace any medical advice or diagnose health issues.

Please note: A lot of the information and ideas expressed in the book come from Homeopathic *Materia Medica* and the author's personal experience.

Please note that products are not to be used as a replacement for homeopathic remedies prescribed by a practitioner.

DEDICATION

TO MY PATIENTS
for the privilege and opportunity to help you
and for the knowledge you taught me.

TO MY MENTORS
for your tireless support, dedication,
comradeship, knowledge, expertise and commitment
to healing humanity and for encouraging me to believe
that the future belongs to those with dreams.

TO ALL THE LIONHEARTS
for the friendship that you gave
that taught me to be brave!

TO MY PARENTS
all honour and praise to the medicine
of my ancestral lineage.

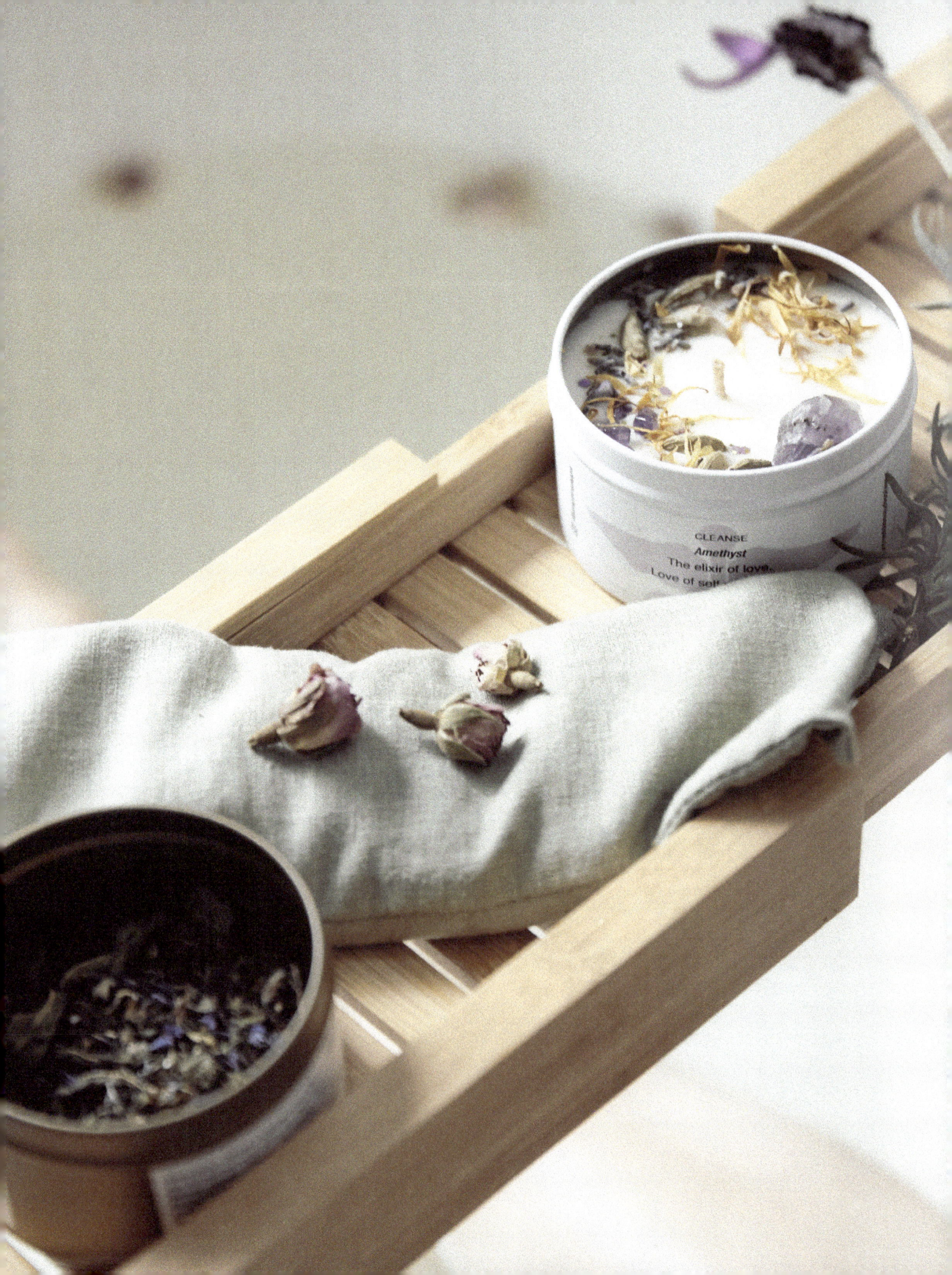

CLEANSE

Amethyst

The elixir of love.
Love of self

CONTENTS

INTRODUCTION
The Soul Contract...

HEAL. (Healing Energy and Love) was created with intention as your destination for healing, wellness products and services. HEAL. is the essence of health; I inspire, empower, and inform people to restore their health through natural therapies and products, with trustworthy, dedicated attention. Homeopathy promotes complete physical, mental and social wellbeing, and nourishes mind, body and soul.

It was my intention to create an offering for people to have an experience with my products. The soul contract already exists and now I am facilitating the energetic visibility of that.

The HEAL. product range was inspired by precious gemstones that carry healing energy and share their gifts with us.

This healing frequency is intended in the range of three extremely unique healing blends that have been created to provide you with the atmospheric essence supportive of effective healing and intent, also supporting cleansing, relaxation, and connection to self.

Homeopathic services are designed to deliver both knowledgeable education and healing with the deep-acting homeopathic remedies prescribed after a consultation.

HEAL. by Josephine is a beginners' guide to homeopathy and is not intended in any way as a full account of *Materia Medica* or prescription advice. This book is designed to create awareness around holistic healthcare and provide alternative offerings for the health-conscious. Homeopathy is a lifelong study and my work in this book only gives a minutia of the available knowledge.

I believe your soul self, the part of you that's always known the way, has led you here. It's time to align with that power within and let it lead the way.

Tune in, every step of the way. My invitation is to use this book as a beautiful, picturesque tabletop book that can be flipped through, and whatever page you land on that particular day is the message for you at that point in time.

So much love from my heart to yours,

Josephine

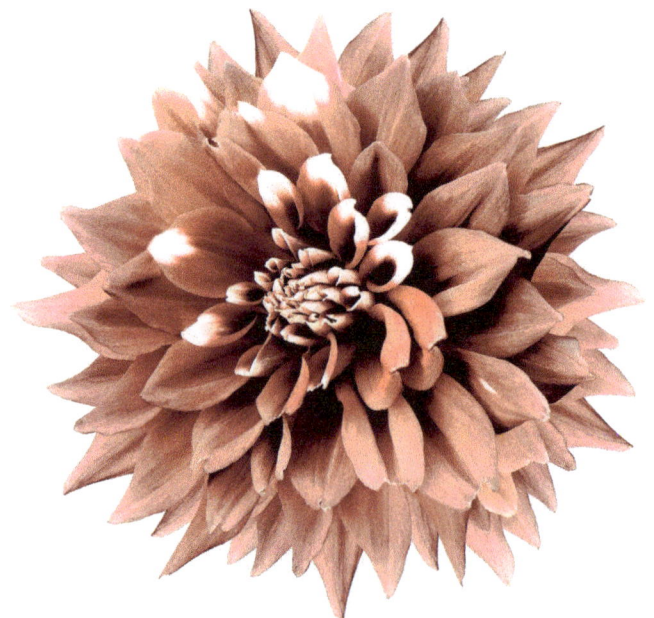

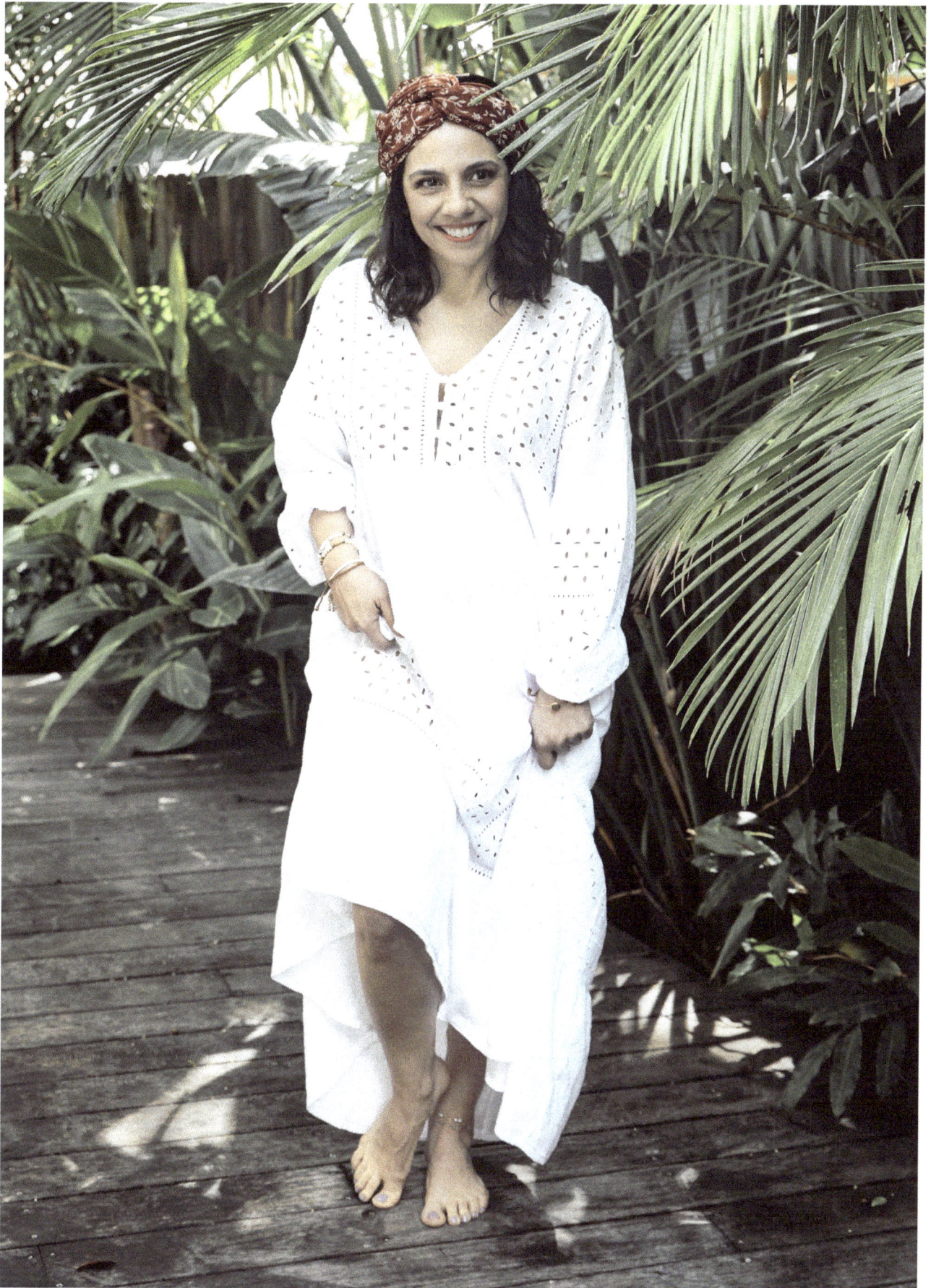

The HEAL. Philosophy

"I expand in abundance, success, and love every day,
as I inspire those around me to do the same."

– Gay Hendricks

Health has always had a significant role in my life. Growing up, food and fresh produce were prioritised, particularly with my family's Italian heritage. Nutrition soon became my passion.

I later went on to study a Bachelor of Health Science, specialising in homeopathic medicine. This of course had the key component of nutrition involved, as nutrition is the foundation of health. Everything you consume either fights disease or feeds it, and nutritional deficiencies create an obstacle to cure when treating homeopathically, as we are not adding anything with homeopathic medicines, we are working *with* what the body already has.

I created HEAL. inspired by the essence of health, to inspire, empower, and inform people to restore their health and nourish their mind, body, and soul. It was formed with intention to be your destination for healing and wellness products and professional services. It's about healing, looking within, aligning your body, and realising your dreams, potential and purpose.

I place a very high emphasis on aligning with the core essence of nature. My ethos, synergies, and brand alignments all align with this. I do not use any single-use plastics throughout the HEAL. range. The herbal tisanes are packaged in biodegradable corn starch cello bags and our cellophane is made from the glucose-polymer, cellulose. It's extracted from natural resources such as wood, cotton, or hemp. Plastic-free, plant-based material.

My work as a writer for health and wellbeing magazines has been featured in *Body & Soul, Balance the Grind, SWIISH, Rescu, Thrive, Green + Simple, Wellbeing, Latte,* and *Brainz.*

I believe we all have the ability to heal ourselves naturally when we work with our body rather than against it.

There is never an emotion without a physical symptom and vice versa. Let it go and let it flow.

Attached to nothing; connected to everything.

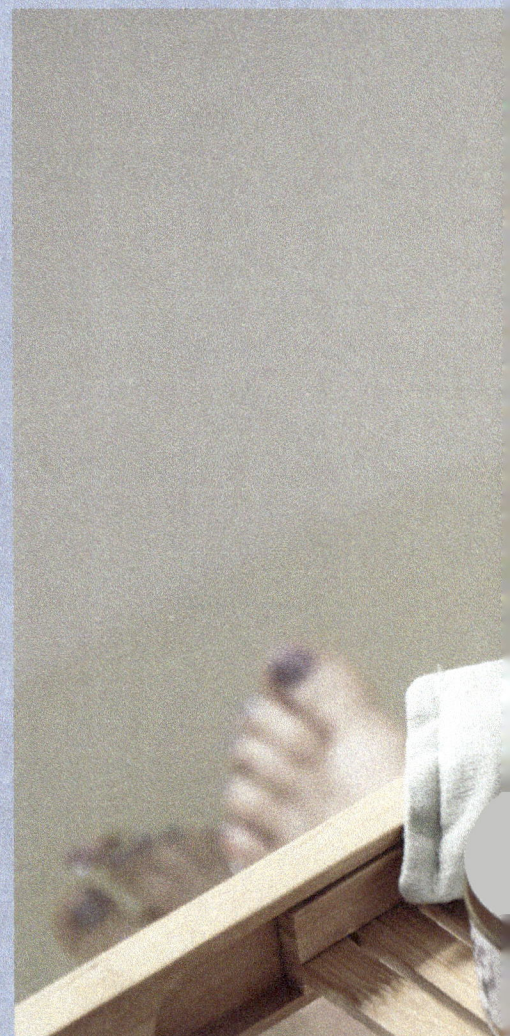

HEAL. products are lovingly handcrafted and packed in Australia and are created with the intention to support cleansing, relaxation and connection to self. The natural ingredients are traditionally used in herbal medicine to purify, calm and support natural healing and intent.

When we dismiss our body's symptoms, we also dismiss our emotions and our own inner guidance. By allowing homeopathy to gently shift the lens through which we operate, we allow our bodies to align back to equilibrium and gently let go of what no longer serves our highest good. Attached to nothing; connected to everything.

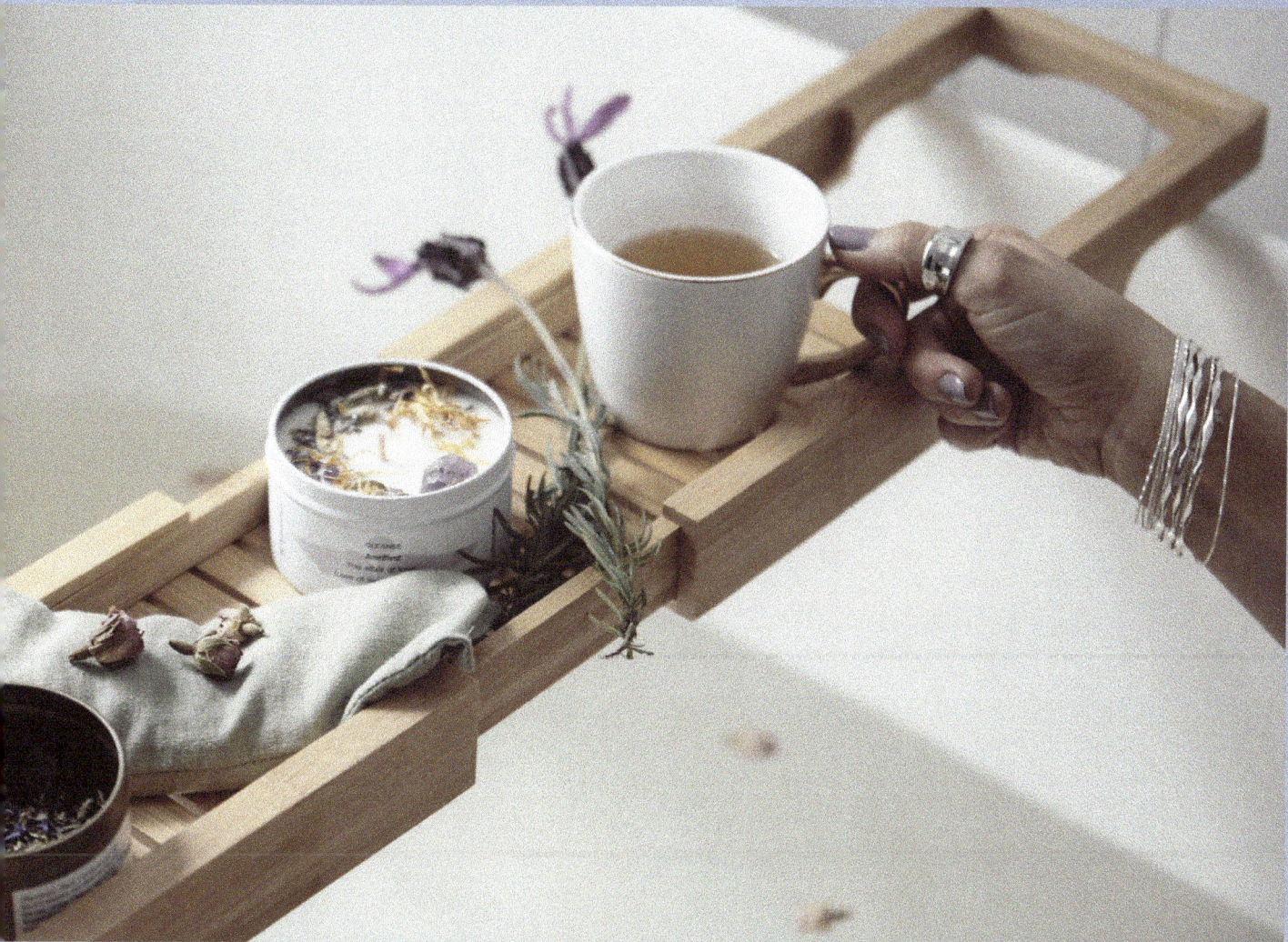

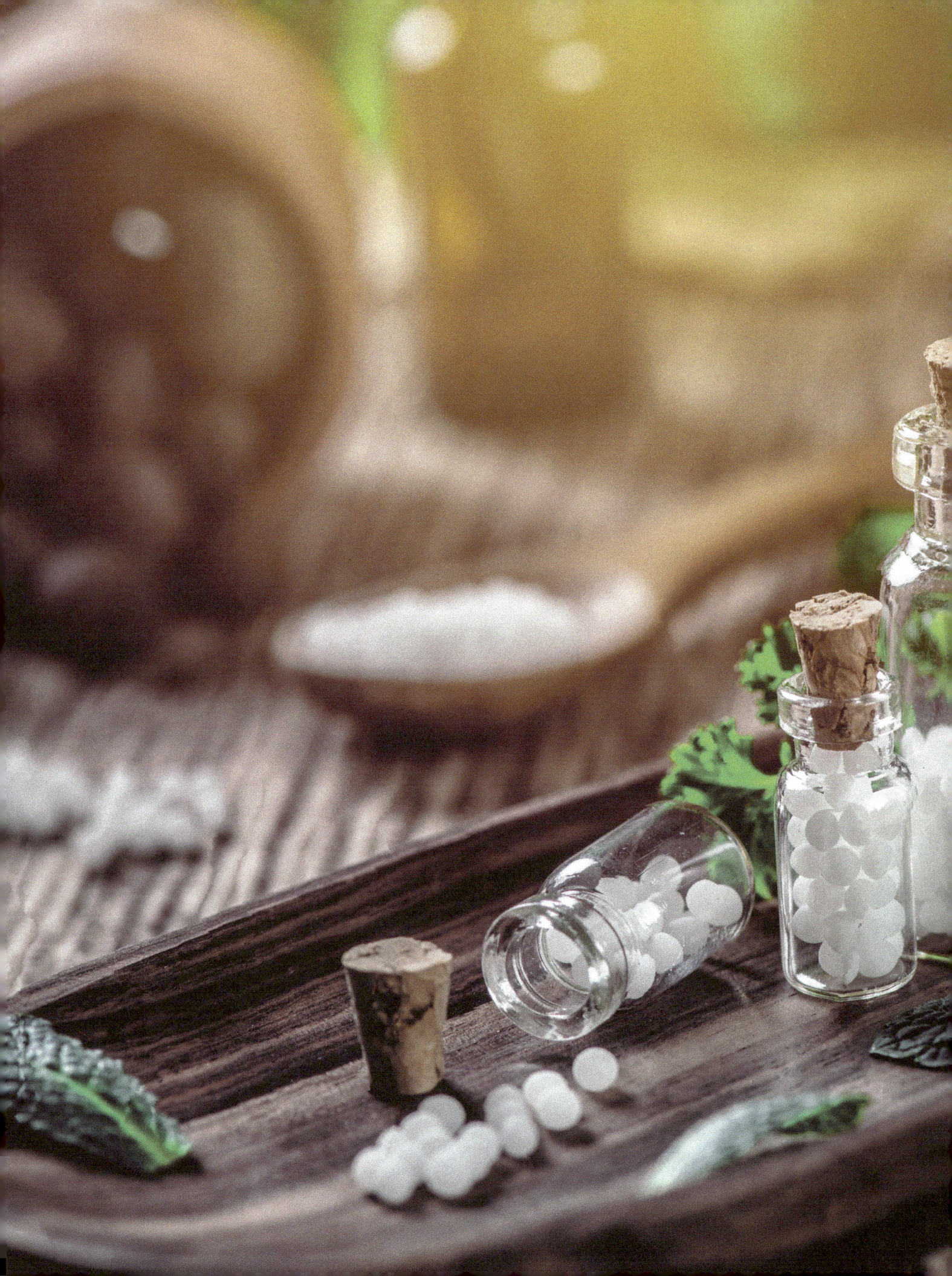

History of homeopathy

What is homeopathy?

Homeopathy has been used for 200 years in most countries around the world. It is used extensively by doctors and practitioners of natural medicine.

Homeopathy was founded by a German doctor, Dr Samuel Hahnemann. Dr Hahnemann was a brilliant physician and pharmacist. Because of his fluency in seven languages, he was able to read healing texts from all communities and all ages.

He was the first physician to make use of the Law of Similars, a Law of Nature known to ancient healers such as Hippocrates. This law states that a substance that is capable of causing a group of symptoms in a healthy person is capable of removing a group of similar symptoms in an unwell person.

Dr Hahnemann realised the value of this law when he was translating a book of medicines from English into German. He disagreed with the author's description of the effects of overdoses of Peruvian Bark, a herb which was used in the treatment of malarial fevers.

Dr Hahnemann, being a true scientist, experimented by taking small doses of the bark and found that he developed a fever that was similar to a malarial fever. The fever stopped when he stopped taking the bark. He took some more, and the fever started again. It stopped soon after he stopped taking the bark.

This was a practical example of the Law of Similars – the bark was capable of producing a fever in a healthy person that was similar to what it could cure in an unwell person.

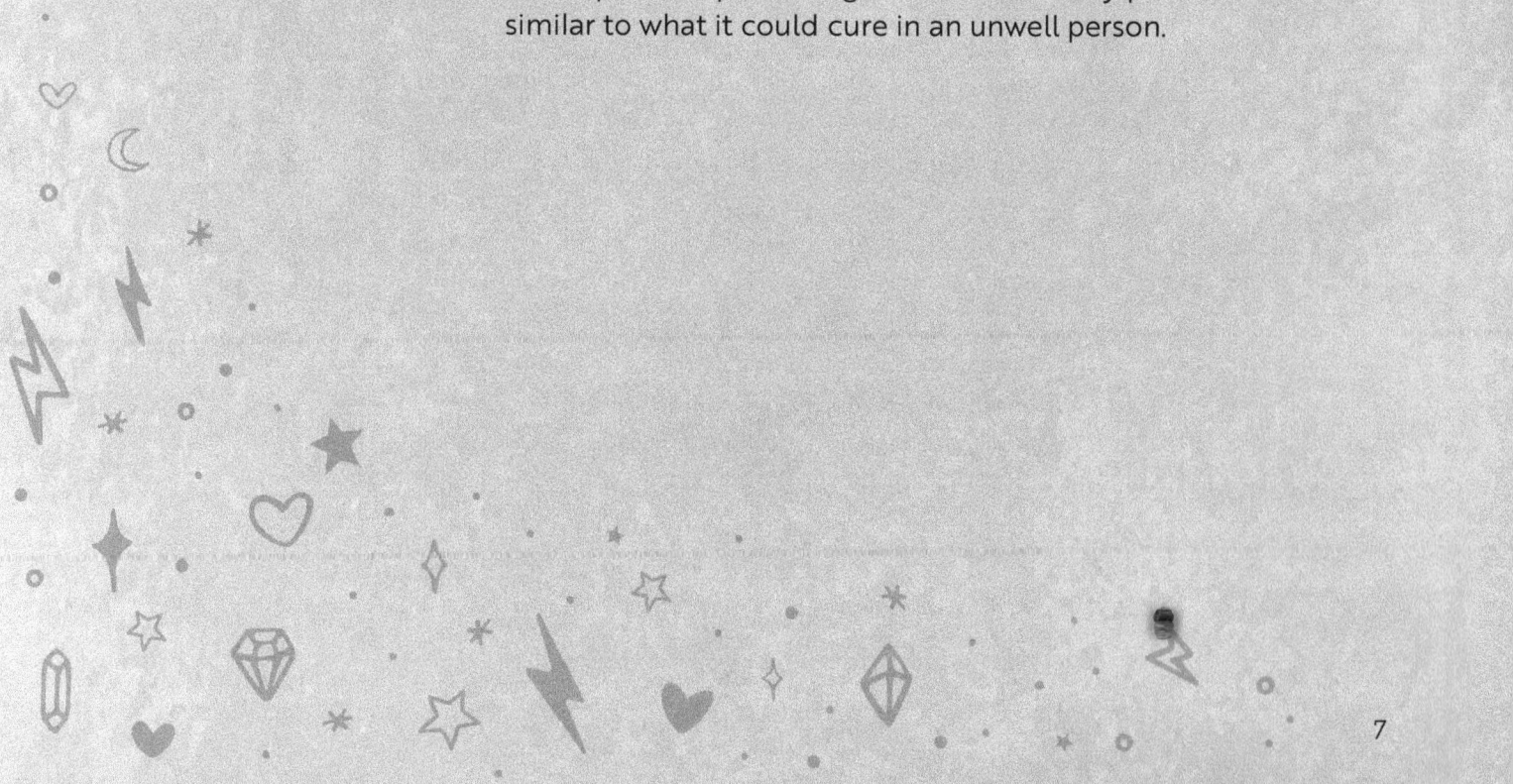

Homeopathy in practice

Over the last 200 years, homeopaths have "proved" thousands of substances. Unlike drug testing, we test our medicines on healthy volunteers who report the resulting symptoms. This is then systematically compiled into a description of what symptoms the substance can remove in unwell patients.

What are homeopathic remedies?

Homeopathic remedies will keep their strength for years without deteriorating. Remedies include carefully selected medicines to treat mental and physical ailments. Medicines should be stored in a cool, dark, dry place with their tops screwed on tightly, well away from strong smelling substances, because strong odours cause the medicines to lose their potency. They should also be stored away from strong light, sun, heat, electrical appliances, strong odours and perfumes (especially camphor, moth balls, menthol and essential oils), and avoid X-rays.

Shake the bottle well before each dose. Medicines should be taken 10-20 minutes before or after anything consumed orally, other than water.

This is so all your delicious mucous membranes can soak up every bit of the medicine without interference from other substances, and you get the best of each dose!

Please note that the patient can have any one of the states described in each homeopathic remedy or nutrition topic. There are many possibilities to bring the symptom picture together and there are many variations of the remedies, so someone needing a particular remedy could be presenting with any of the states that are described. Throughout this book, many state and symptom possibilities will be outlined.

Please note: Products are not to be used as a replacement for homeopathic remedies prescribed by a practitioner.

We get to a point
in our lives where
we're not sick and
we call that 'health',
but we have so much
more potential.

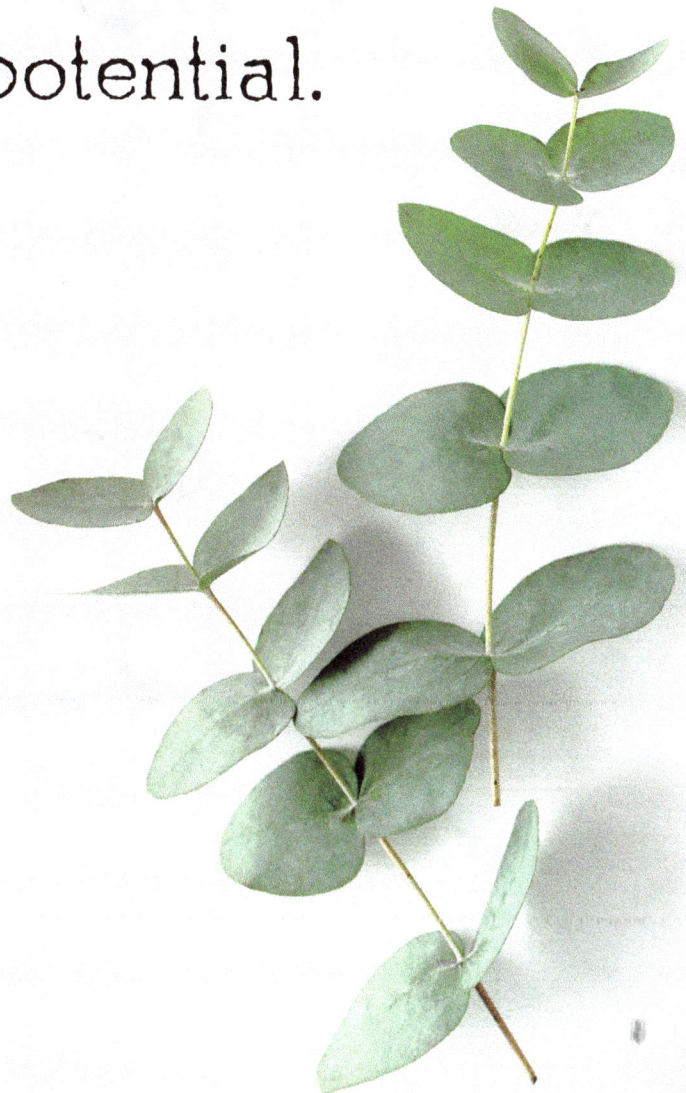

HEAL. candles, oils and teas

The candles and healing oils have been designed with intention for my patients with skin sensitivities and allergies, and created to provide you with an atmospheric essence supportive of effective healing and intent. They are perfect for meditations, yoga, romance, new or full moon intention setting, and during skincare, night-time and bath rituals. Burn candles for no more than three hours at a time. Always keep candles in sight when in use; always burn candles in a well-ventilated room. The candle, container and wax can become hot when in use.

The teas are soothing, hydrating and healing tisanes created to support cleansing, relaxation and connection to self. Steep one teaspoon per cup of freshly boiled water for three to five minutes and allow the ingredients to mature and liberate the aroma. Store in a cool dry place.

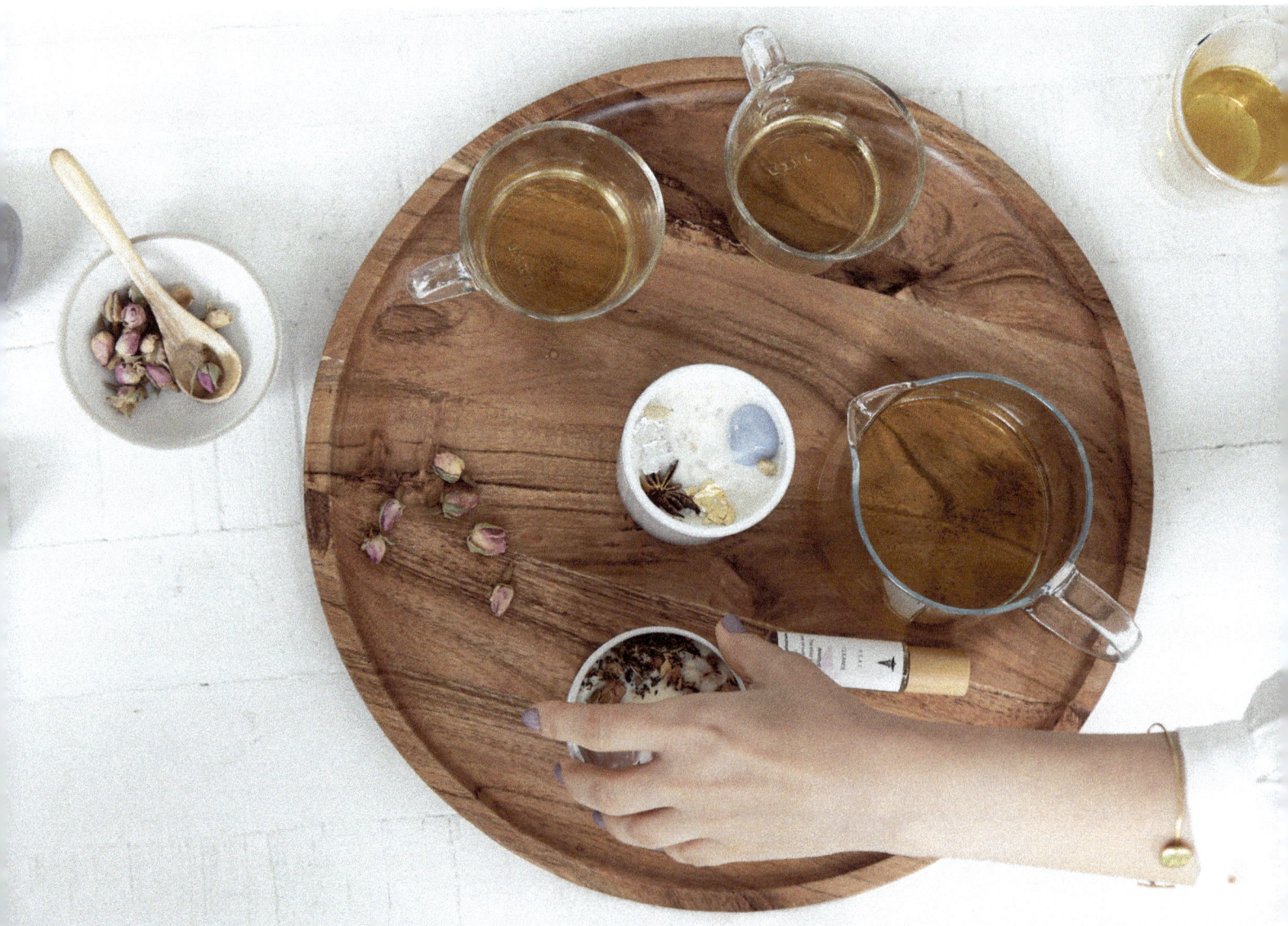

Terminology

This section will give some context to homeopathic language used in this book.

Firstly, to me, healing means aligning body, mind, soul and spirit. It can mean healing the mind of a long-held belief that no longer serves you. Healing is not merely the absence of disease or infirmity.

✧ 'Clinical symptoms' refer to what we will often see in clinic when talking to a patient or when investigating the patient's medical history, rather than what we see from giving the remedy or the symptoms we use as guidance to prescribe the remedy.

✧ 'Contraindicated' refers to situations where there is a condition that means the treatment should not be undertaken because it could cause harm.

✧ 'Genetic' refers to family history and inherited genes that predispose to a specific condition.

✧ 'Indications' or 'indicated' means that a particular treatment is suitable in the situation.

✧ 'Keynotes' are the guiding symptoms for the homeopathic remedy.

✧ 'Miasm' (in homeopathic literature) refers to the hereditary predisposition, which is deeper than a genetic cause. Miasms can include genetic predispositions to disease, but they are not limited to the specific disease's condition. The inherited miasmatic picture expresses through the genetic specific condition and could be any of the fundamental miasms requiring treatment. Samuel Hahnemann, the German physician who founded homeopathy, referred to it as the 'miasmatic taint'. For example, hayfever is an allergic hypersensitivity from the same family as asthma and atopic eczema; hayfever is the miasmatic expression of the disease.

✧ 'Negative and positive essences': There are two sides or polarities to every remedy. There is a negative essence and a positive essence – and it is the same with people; we are either up or down. Remedies help align the patient, bringing them back to equilibrium without being stuck in either. This is health in its greatest form.

✧ 'Nosodes' are homeopathic remedies prepared from human diseased tissue.

✧ 'Provings' are how homeopathic remedies and immersions are tested.

✧ 'Provers' are volunteers in clinical studies.

✧ 'Psychosomatic' means that it reflects the interconnection between psyche, mind, and soma (body).

✧ 'Sarcodes' are homeopathic remedies prepared from healthy human tissue and secretions.

PRODUCTS

Alternative offerings for the health-conscious

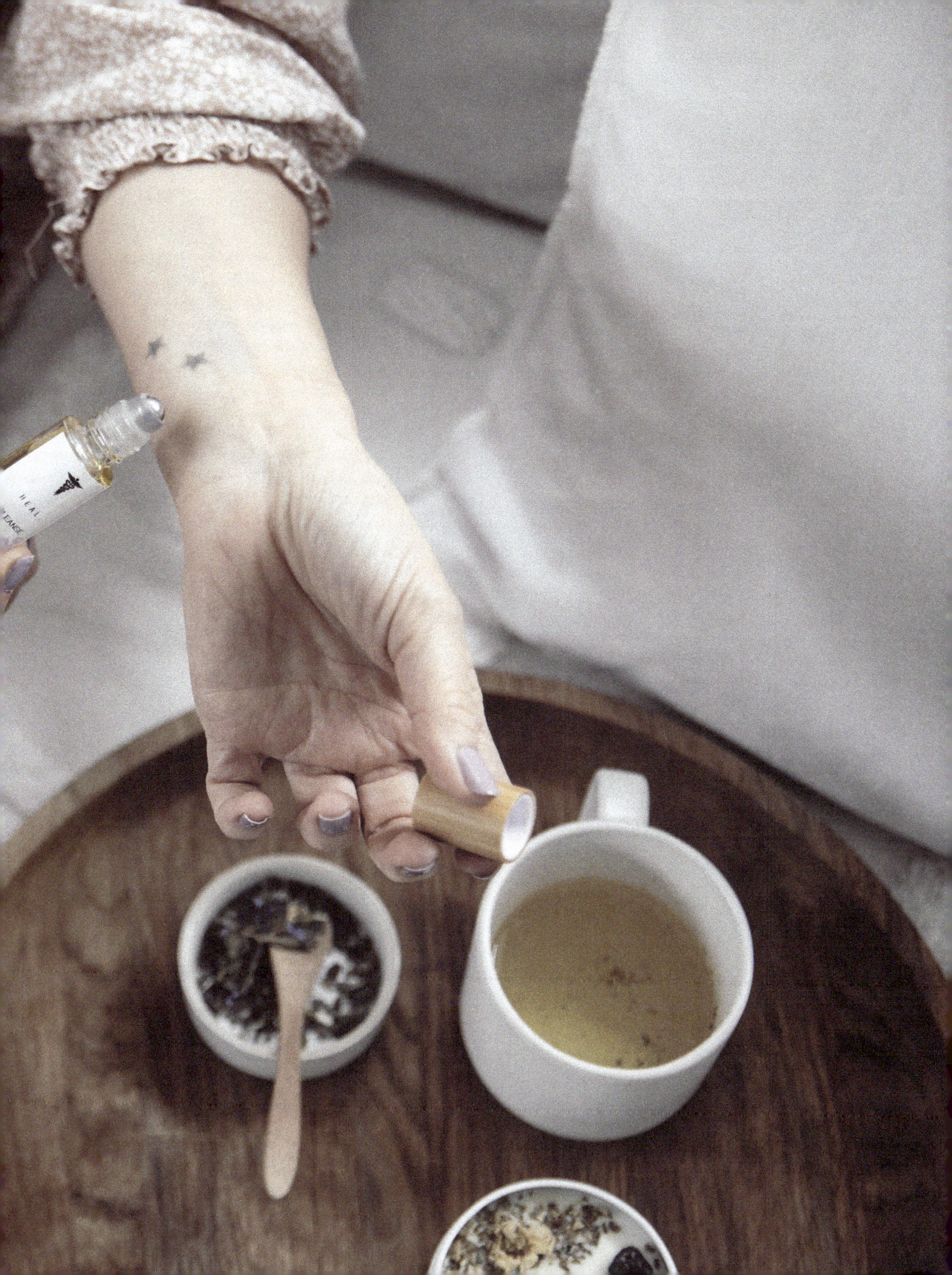

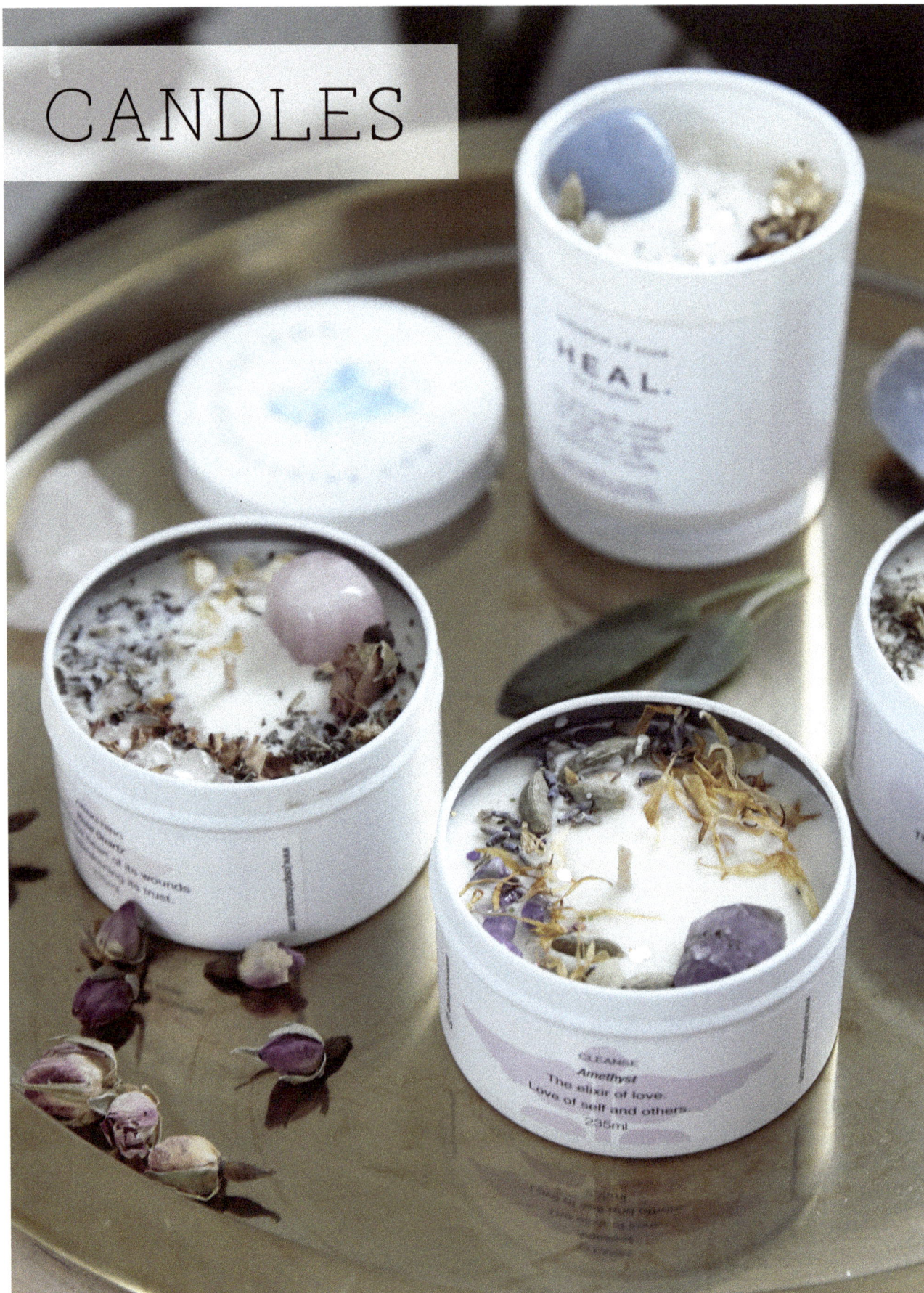

CANDLES

CLEANSE
Amethyst
The elixir of love.
Love of self and others
235ml

Rose Quartz / Awakening

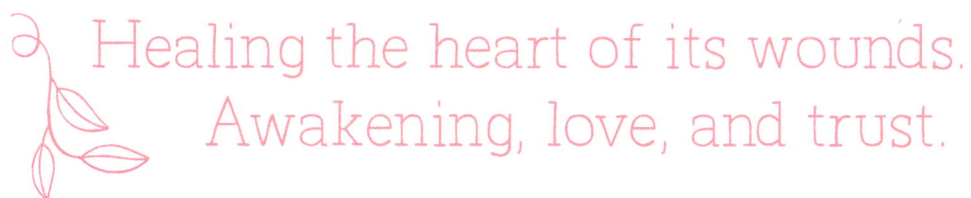

Healing the heart of its wounds.
Awakening, love, and trust.

Rose Quartz Crystal: Universal stone of love, restores trust and harmony in relationships. Encourages self-love and also love for others, helps to heal wounding related to the father or the masculine principle. Opens the heart to giving, receiving, and sharing, calms aggression, resentment, balances and strengthens the heart and emotions, supports compassion, forgiveness, patience. Rose Quartz opens the heart for inner healing, peace, and romance. Also known as a fertility crystal, Rose Quartz catalyses the opportunity to birth new life, rebirth yourself, your hope and trust, and in doing so heal your unloved parts.

Rose Quartz is composed of silica giving an array of exquisite rose pink tones.

It is a healing tool for those hurt by love, enhancing feelings of compassion for those we love, including ourselves.

Affirmation:
I open my heart to receive
and express the energy of love.

INGREDIENTS

Crystal
Rose Quartz

Pure essential oils
Lavender: Cleansing mind, body, spirit, eases stress and anxiety, purity, devotion, resonates with the crown chakra and the Violet Ray of Transmutation.

Patchouli: Heals feelings of loss, separation, abandonment, isolation. Patchouli is also known for the properties of prosperity, spiritual growth, passion, fertility, beauty.

Ylang-ylang: Sensuality, emotional healing, nourishes the heart, heals deep emotional trauma.

Jasmine: Attracts love, romantic, spiritual, and unconditional. It also supports purification, healing, self-confidence. Associated with the Moon it supports women's cycles.

Sweet orange: Acceptance, focus, known for its power to uplift mood, promote healing.

Botanicals
Jasmine: Attracts love, romantic, spiritual, and unconditional. It also supports purification, healing, self-confidence. Associated with the Moon, it supports women's cycles.

Rose: Attunement, strengthens and balances the heart, universal symbol of love, sacred flower to goddesses throughout history.

Lavender: Cleansing mind, body spirit, eases stress and anxiety, purity, devotion, connects the heart with the crown chakra.

Chamomile: Chamomile is the botanical of manifestation, abundance and purification, attracting love and calming fiery emotions.

Peppermint: Peppermint inspires purification, healing, psychic powers, love and connection.

Lemon balm: Lemon balm activates healing, love, success, releasing and longevity.

DISCOVER THIS
PRODUCT

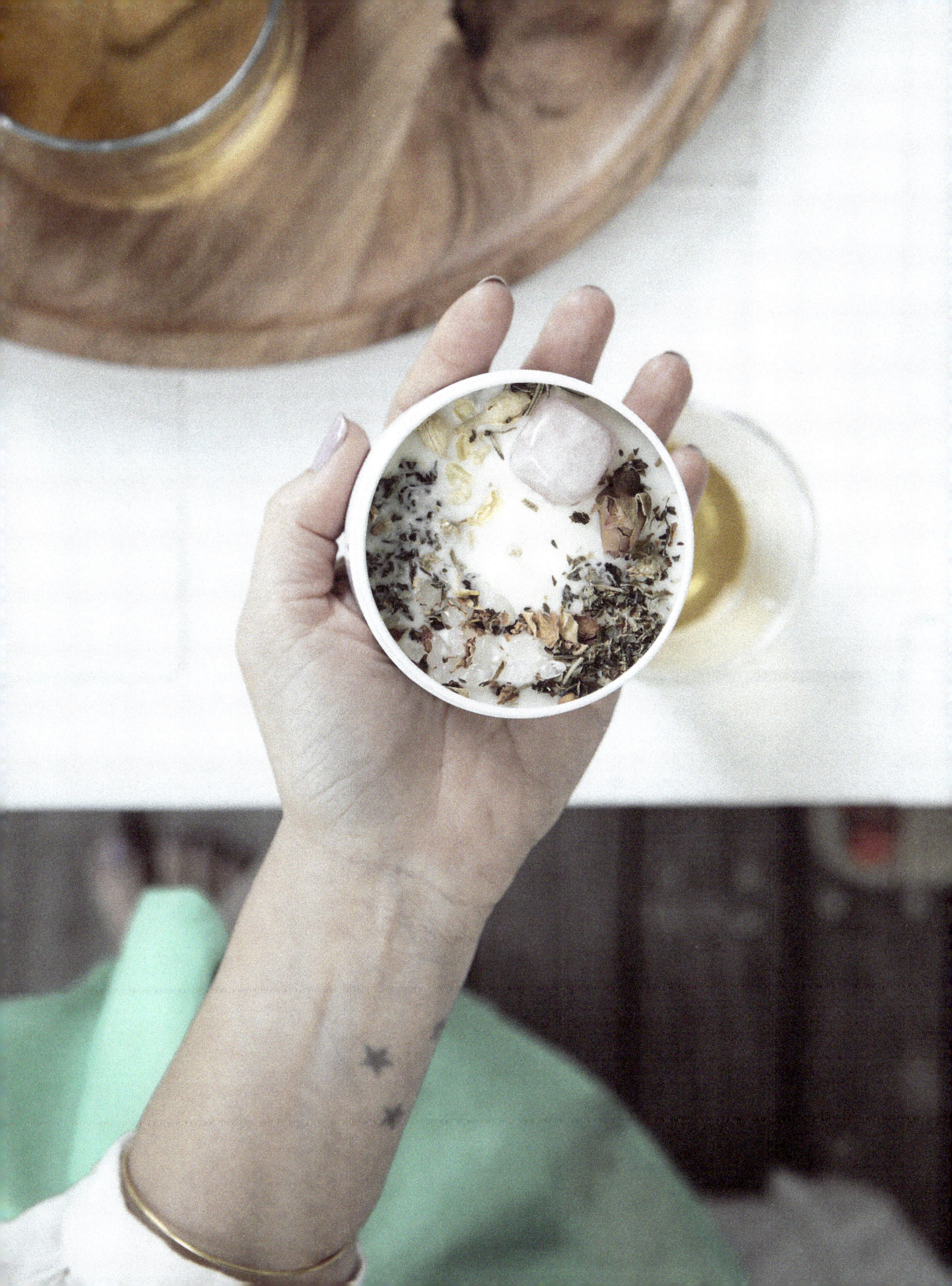

Amethyst / Cleanse

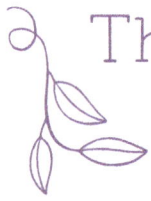

The essence of love, purification, and divine connection.

Amethyst crystal stimulates protection, purification and divine connection.

Amethyst opens and clears the third eye and crown chakras; it accelerates the development of intuition, psychic abilities and mindfulness.

Amethyst is a crystal of physical healing. It is believed to aid memory, coordinates the brain with the nervous system, transmutes and dissolves negativity (such as grief, anxiety, rage, fear and stress) and exposes the root causes of behavioural and emotional patterns so they can be worked on.

Amethyst is silicon dioxide with properties of the quartz group of minerals. It instigates the ability and desire to see yourself as you are, taking you outside the limits of your everyday perception. It enables you to identify mental, emotional and behavioural baggage and promotes the desire to resolve it, to 'cleanse' mentally and physically.

This gemstone crystal is the essence of love; love of self and others. Its energy infuses into you and emanates into the way you communicate and connect in your relationships.

This violet-coloured stone is perfect to sit by your bedside to promote complete alignment with the mental and spiritual self.

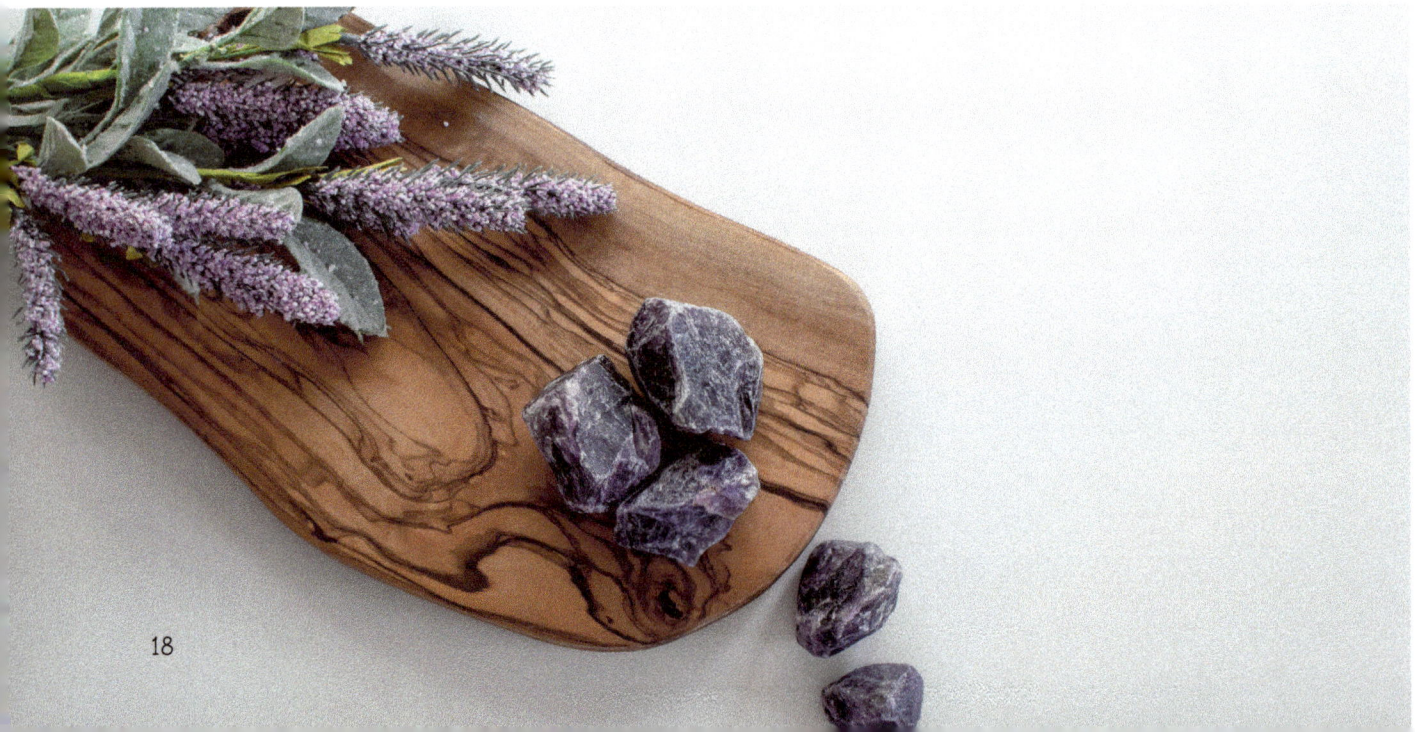

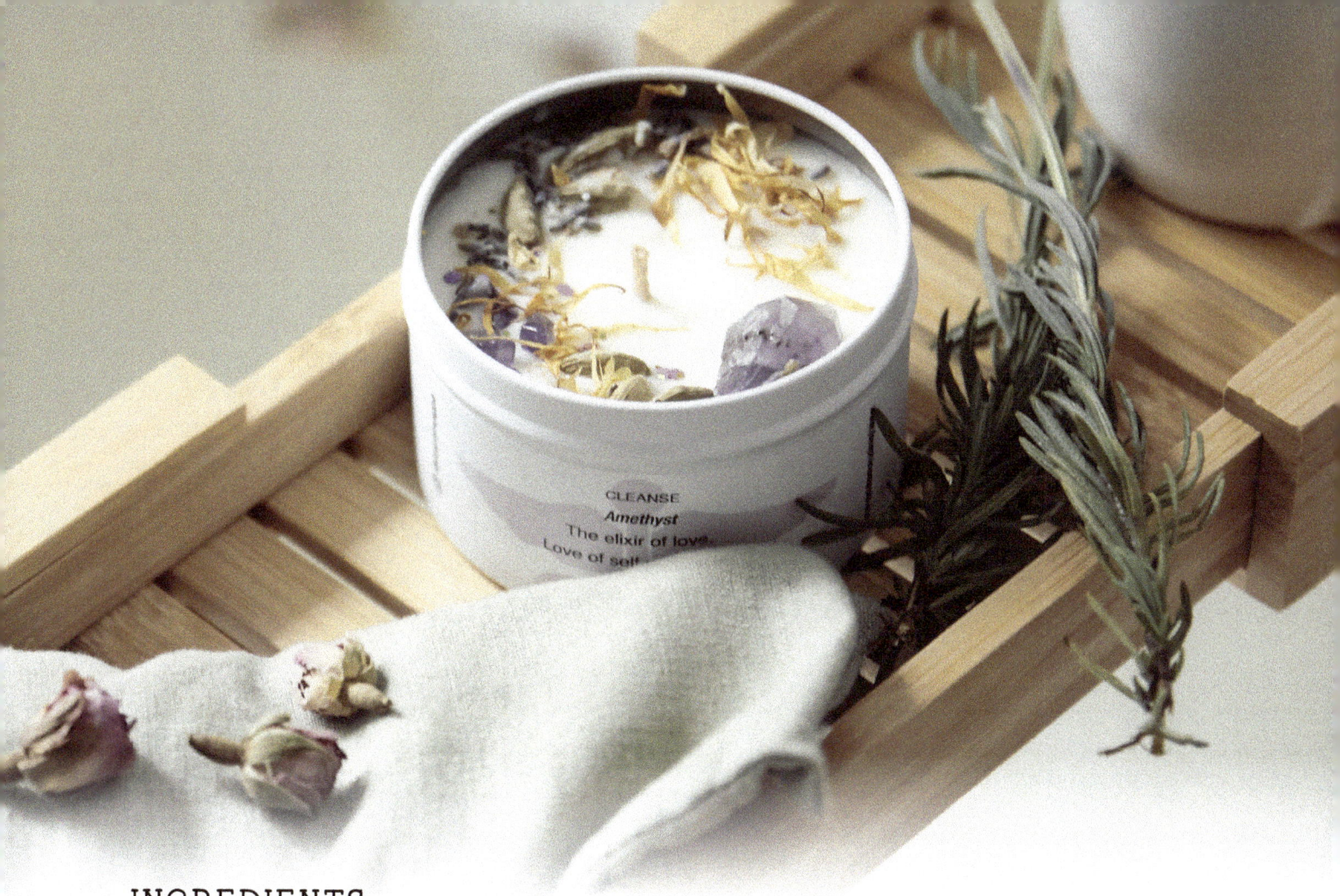

INGREDIENTS

Crystal
Amethyst

Pure essential oils
Grapefruit: Grapefruit cleanses aura and mental body and clears mental chatter.

Lemon: Lemon stimulates balance and strength, and awakens the third eye.

Bergamot: Bergamot relieves stress, grief and depression and drives stability.

Cardamom: Cardamom encourages love, sensuality, spiritual awakening, insight and wisdom.

Sage: Sage is the herb of protection, clearing, purification and ritual.

Botanicals
Calendula: Calendula represents healing, with soothing and antiseptic properties.

Cardamom: Cardamom improves anxiety, encourages healing, and is considered a sacred plant in Eastern cultures.

Lavender: Lavender cleanses mind, body and spirit and eases stress and anxiety. It encourages purity and devotion and resonates with the crown chakra.

DISCOVER THIS PRODUCT

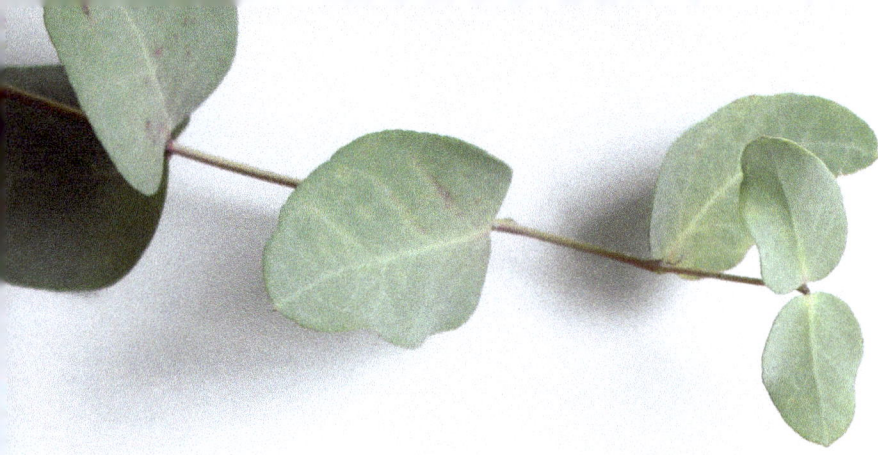

We have a soul contract to have an experience together through my products or services. This contract already exists and now I am facilitating the energetic visibility of that.

Connect in with my intention, the energy of my offerings, and to the shift you're going to experience with that.

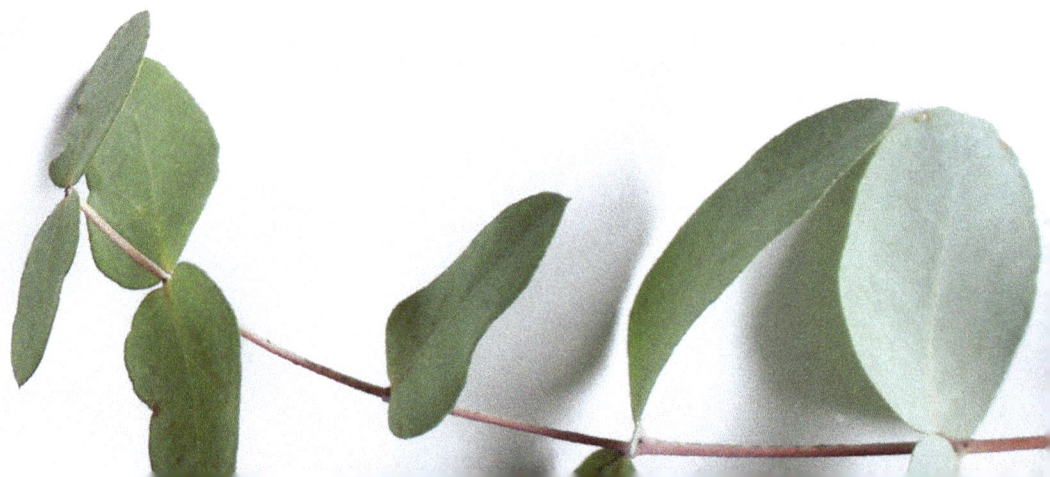

☪ ♡ ♥

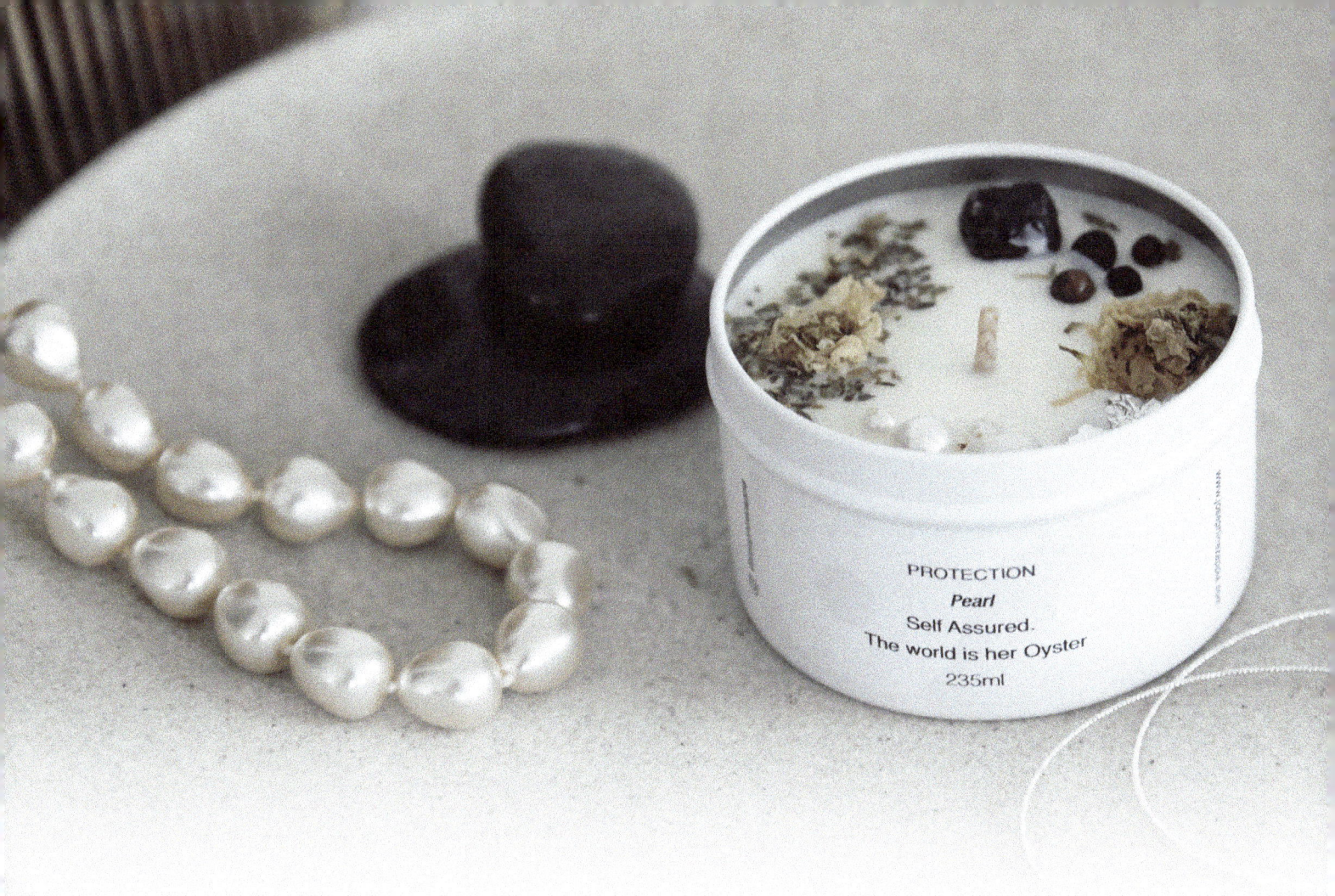

Pearl / Protection

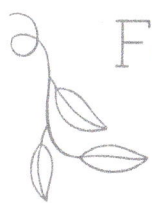

Feminine powers of wisdom, nurturing, and intuition. Powers of the mystical moon and purification.

Just like the oyster takes the sand and turns it into a beautiful pearl, we too have the ability to alchemise discomfort, stuck energy, emotional imbalances and turn it into courage, knowingness, and strength. Just as the distinctive protective power of the (oyster) shell is ingrained in the pearl itself, so is this knowingness within us.

Pearl represents wisdom gained through experience, luck and wealth, purity and integrity. It encourages nurturing actions and soothes and heals negativity.

Seen as the symbol of femininity, patience, strength and power, pearls are associated with the powers of the mystical moon, water cycles and divine light connected to spirit.

Physically pearls are believed to aid muscular system conditions, pain and discomfort during childbirth and digestive disorders.

INGREDIENTS

Crystals
Pearl

Black tourmaline: Black tourmaline has the ability to purify negative energy, to protect one's energy fields and release attachments. It has a strong grounding force and powerful energy supporting transformation. Black tourmaline helps one to create and hold protective boundaries, both emotionally and physically.

Pure essential oils
Lavender: Lavender cleanses mind, body and spirit and eases stress and anxiety. It encourages purity and devotion and resonates with the crown chakra, and has a connection to the higher mind.

Ylang-ylang: Ylang-ylang encourages sensuality and emotional healing. It nourishes the heart, and aids in healing deep emotional trauma.

Frankincense: Frankincense is healing and soothing. It lifts the vibration in the body, purifies and releases inflammation.

Cedarwood atlas: Cedarwood atlas is extremely grounding and balancing, supporting meditative states of consciousness.

Sandalwood: Cleansing and calming, sandalwood has a high vibrational frequency, making it a powerful aid in supporting manifestation and all creative endeavours.

Carrier oil: Camelia.

Botanicals
Chrysanthemum flowers: Chrysanthemum flowers signify balance, loyalty, devotion, love, longevity and joy.

Juniper berries: Juniper berries denote protection, ritual, magic and purification.

Passionflower: Passionflower encourages passion and spirituality, promotes stress release, and aids joy and lightheartedness.

DISCOVER THIS PRODUCT

Initiation of Trust

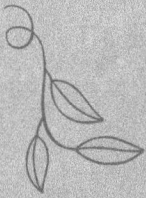

Angelite crystal aids contact with the angelic realms, your spirit guides, and light beings in the higher spiritual realms. This crystal stimulates the birth of psychic gifts such as clairvoyance, mental telepathy, channelling, mediumship and automatic writing. It helps one cope with difficult emotional situations, calming and soothing tension, stress, and anger.

INGREDIENTS

Clear quartz chips: In mythology, clear quartz is valued by many civilisations as far back as Lemuria and was used extensively in Atlantis. In the metaphysical world, clear quartz is believed to be the ultimate healer, balancing and revitalising the physical, mental, emotional, and spiritual bodies, as well as stimulating the immune system and restoring the body back into perfect balance.

Clear quartz amplifies whatever energy or intent is programmed into it, and when placed with other crystals or gemstones, it also amplifies their energy and metaphysical properties.

Its ruling planet is the sun, and it resonates with all four elements – water, earth, fire and air. It primarily resonates with the crown chakra, but it is also used to balance the entire chakra system.

Star anise: Star anise is rich in antioxidant and anti-inflammatory properties. Its spiritual attributes are purification, protection, divination, psychic awareness, cleansing and fertility.

Gold: Gold leaf is used in the candle to support the balancing of the masculine and feminine principle. Gold is believed to inspire virtue and moral excellence, positive attitudes, thinking and growth. It has long been associated with the sun and the element of fire and is believed to open one up to wisdom. Gold is said to increase the healing power of crystals and gemstones. The high priests in many ancient cultures, including Egypt, Mesopotamia, and Greece, understood this and how to work with crystals and gemstones. They fashioned ceremonial tools and breastplates from gold, gemstones and crystals to enhance their status and power. Gold also represents the divine masculine force within each of us, which can connote balance, action and manifestation.

Keywords:

Attunement

Healing

Amplification

Acceleration

Clarity

Balance

Revitalisation

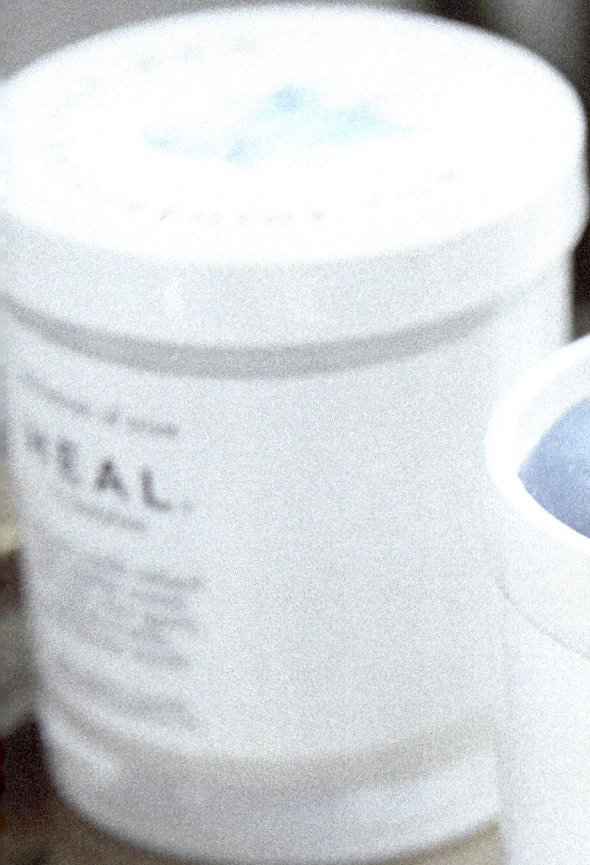

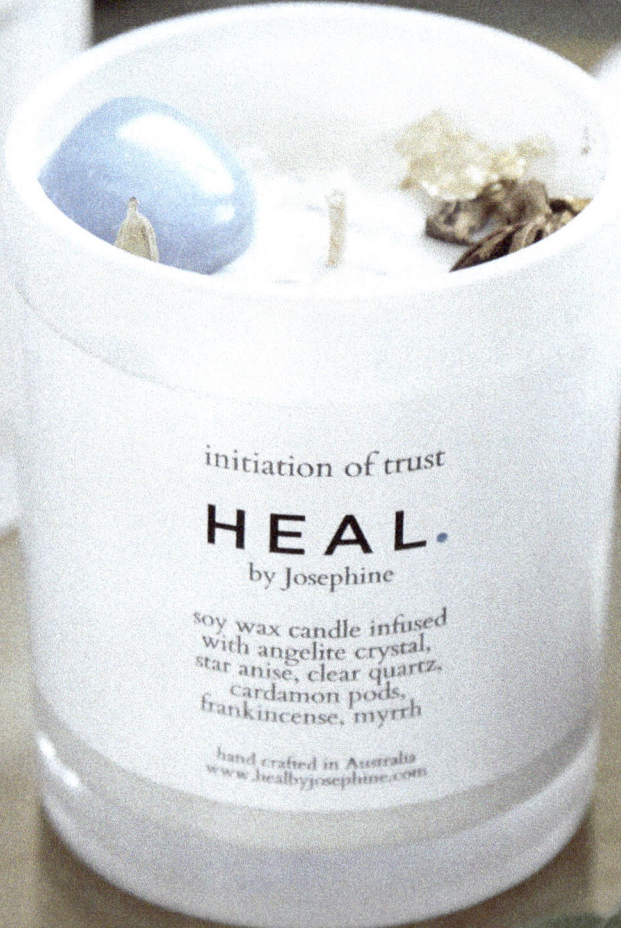

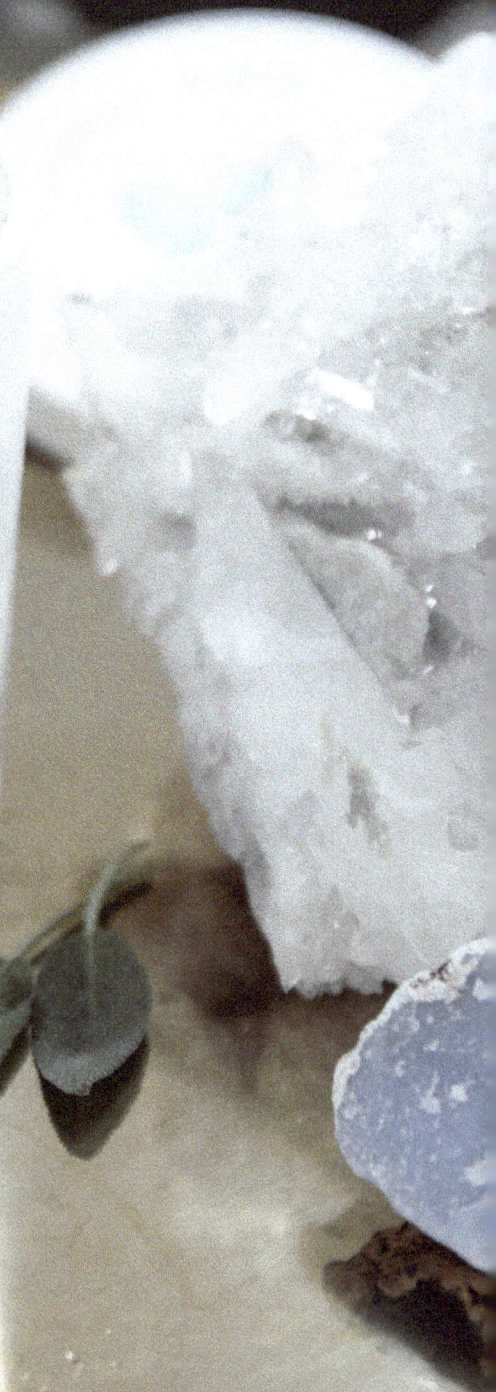

initiation of trust

HEAL.

by Josephine

soy wax candle infused
with angelite crystal,
star anise, clear quartz,
cardamon pods,
frankincense, myrrh

hand crafted in Australia
www.healbyjosephine.com

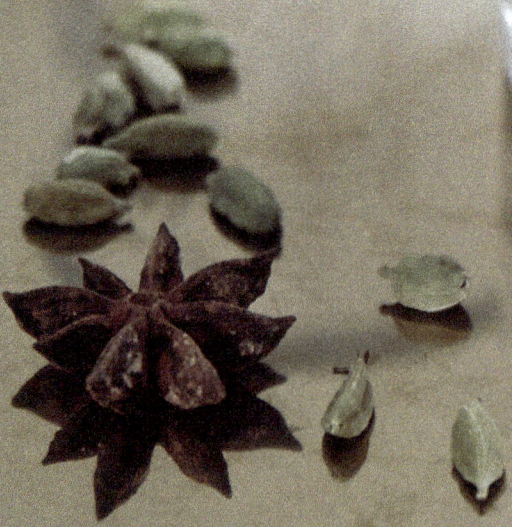

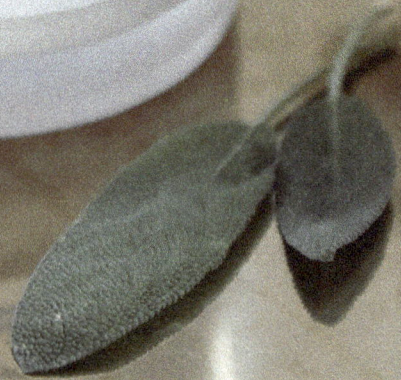

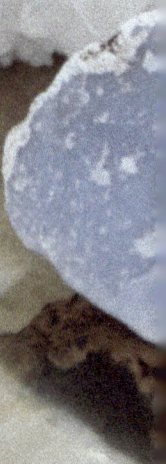

Silver: Silver leaf has also been incorporated into the candle. It is associated with the moon goddess. It is a receptive feminine energy, and is soft but strong, as well as nurturing and creative. It resonates with the element of water.

Silver helps one attune to the lunar frequencies and the flow of the universe. It is the metal of the emotions, love and healing, and its energies are stronger during astrological alignments involving the moon, or on new or full moons. The properties associated with silver are manifestation of wealth and health, enhancement, creativity, enhanced communication, balance, and serenity. Silver also represents the divine feminine principle within each of us.

Stars: The stars were added to the candle to represent the universal cosmic forces and their link to the earth's planetary forces. The phrase "as above, so below" reminds us of our origins and our connection to the cosmos. There are many spiritual meanings behind stars – they are symbols of the deity and the highest achievements spiritually. They also symbolise divine guidance and protection; they were known to represent miracles. The Star card in the Tarot deck represents love, hope, relationships and romance. Stars also symbolise humanity, faith, excellence, motivation, magic and truth. They are typically tied to inspiration, aspiration, imagination, pursuits and dreams.

Cardamom: Cardamom is known for its extraordinary healing powers. It is also known for its spiritual qualities and is used in ceremonies as offerings to Hindu gods and goddesses, as it is believed to stimulate one's inner wisdom and the inner spiritual senses. Cardamom also helps one to let go of feelings of unworthiness that keep one from achieving goals and desires. Its other effects include opening the heart and stimulating the feelings of love, as well as facilitating the releasing of attachments and letting go of burdens, fears and worries.

Pure essential oils
Frankincense and Myrrh oil
Lavender Oil

Keywords:

Heightened perception and understanding

Creativity

Emotional strength

Strengthening of the astral body

Intuition

DISCOVER THIS PRODUCT

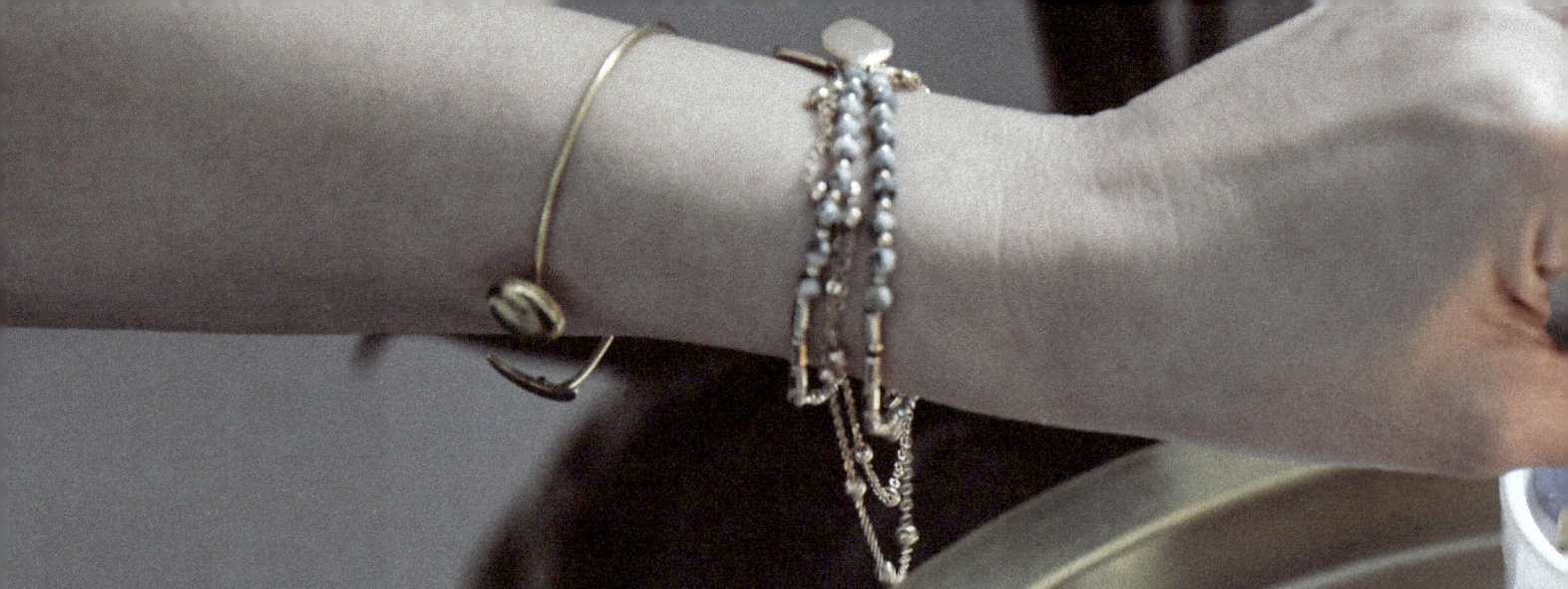

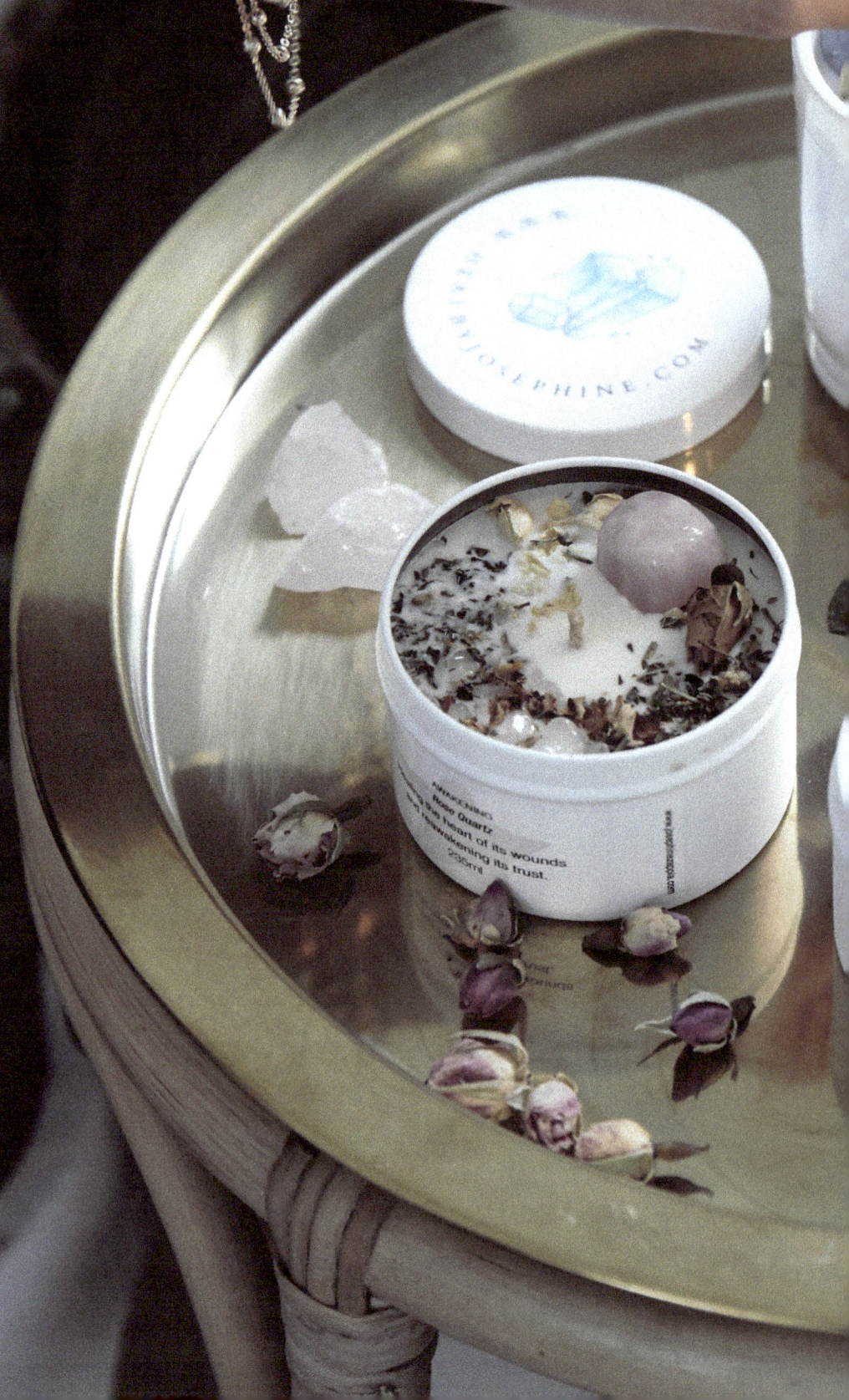

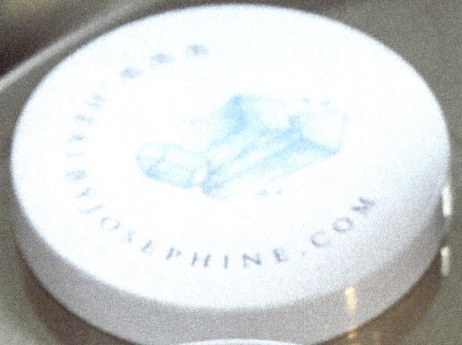

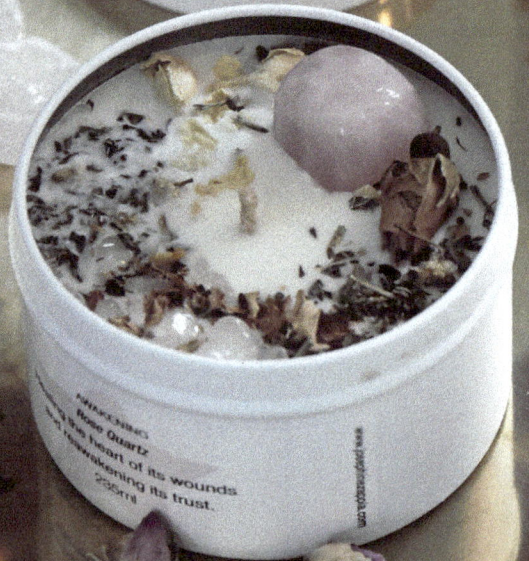

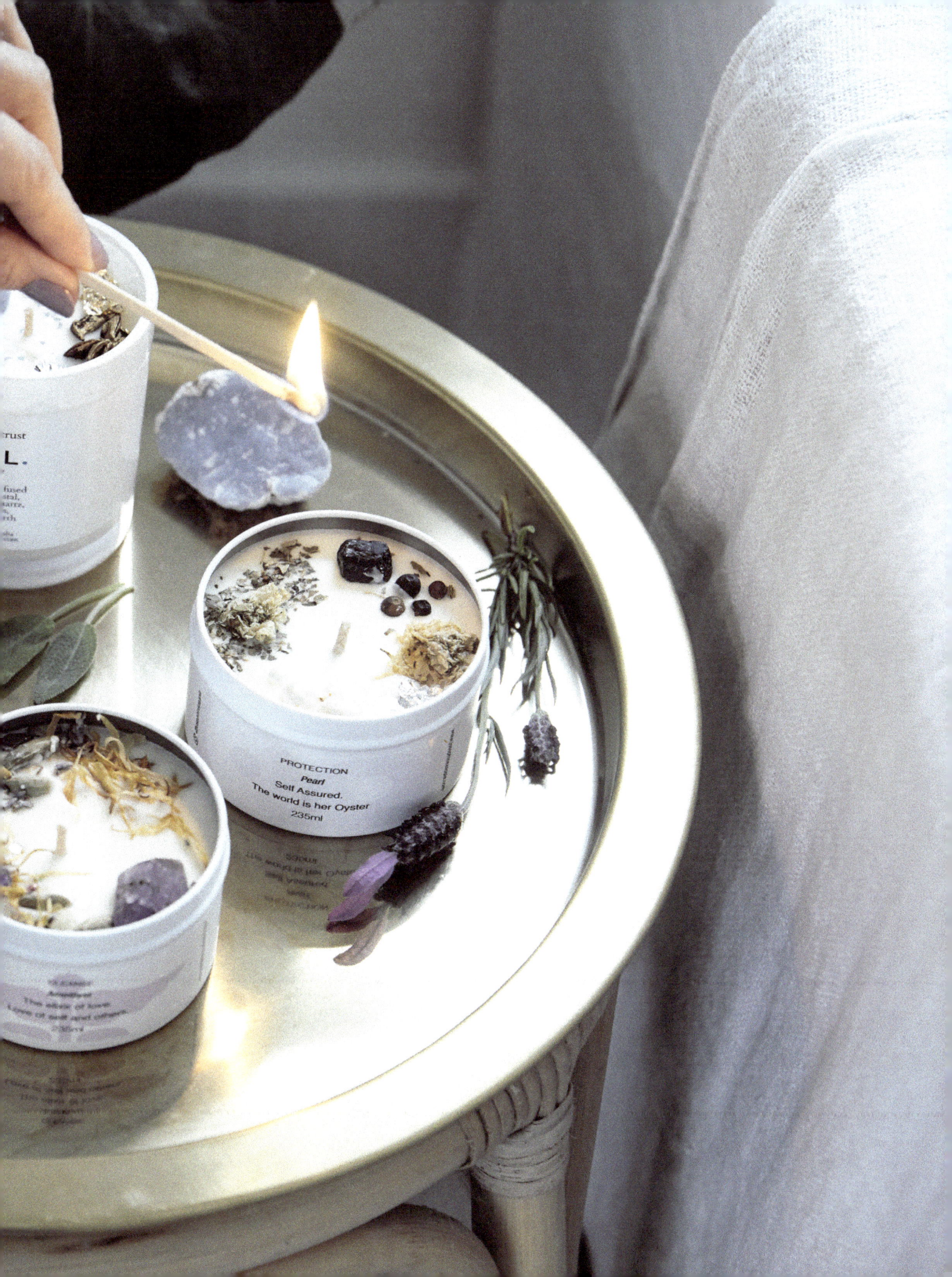

L.

rust

fused
stal,
arre,
rth

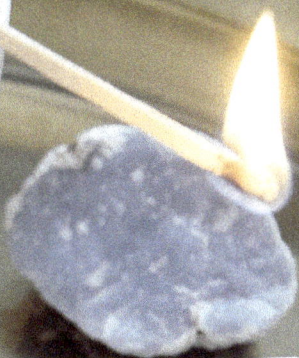

PROTECTION
Pearl
Self Assured.
The world is her Oyster
235ml

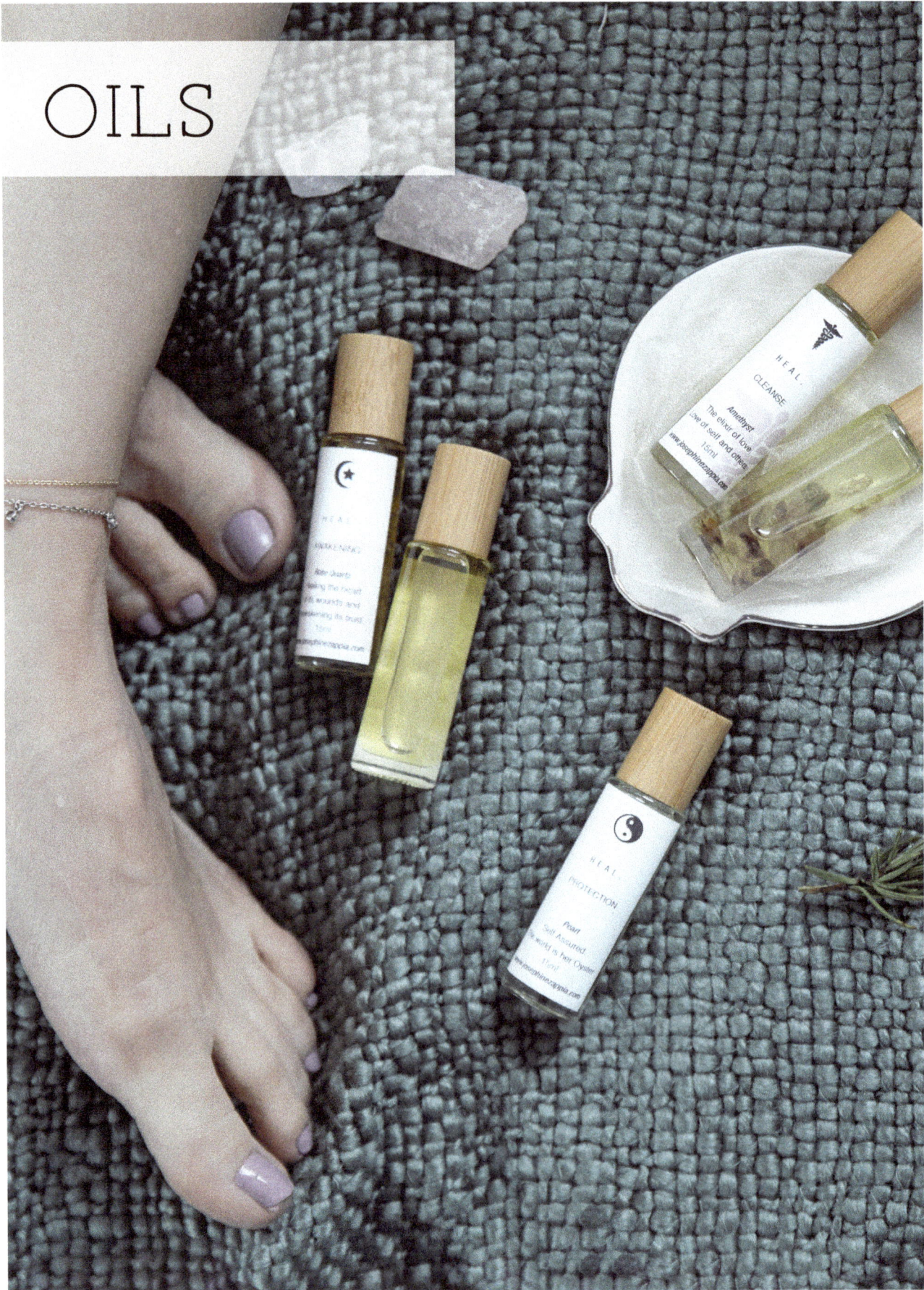

OILS

About the oils

The oils were inspired into creation for my patients with skin sensitivities and allergies, who are very attuned to touch, sound and smell through every sense of our body, HEAL. has a range of distinctively individual fragrance oils: Pearl, Amethyst and Rose Quartz.

HEAL. pure essential oil blends are handmade can be used as a body scent or perfume. They are gentle and non-irritating to sensitive skin and allergies.

As with our healing candle range, our fragrance oils are extraordinary, unique and designed with intention. The three healing blends have been thoughtfully created to provide you with the purest, natural, ritualistic self-care products that hold a healing frequency and support natural healing and intent.

Each of the fragrant oils have a divine blend of premium essential oils, with Jojoba as the carrier oil, and a small gemstone (Pearl, Amethyst or Rose Quartz) within it to further support the healing and intention-setting ritual. They are in a 15mL bamboo glass roller bottle and can be applied to pulse points.

Mind and body always speak the same language. So a patient who is so oversensitive physically is also going to be over sensitive and reactive mentally.

Also expressing as overly anxious and stressed.

Rose Quartz / Awakening

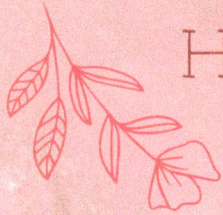

Healing the heart of its wounds.
Awakening, love, and trust.

The Rose Quartz roll-on is a blend of Lavender, Patchouli, Ylang-ylang, Jasmine and Sweet orange. You can apply the oil to your pulse points. The roller bottle also contains Rose Quartz crystals to enhance and energise the heart chakra and the essential oils.

DISCOVER THIS
PRODUCT

Affirmation:
I open my heart to receive
and express the energy of love.

INGREDIENTS

Gemstone
Rose Quartz

Pure essential oils

Lavender: Lavender helps to cleanse the mind, body and spirit, eases stress and anxiety, and symbolises purity and devotion. It resonates with the crown chakra and the Violet Ray of Transmutation.

Patchouli: Patchouli works to heal feelings of loss, separation, abandonment and isolation. Patchouli is also known for the properties of prosperity, spiritual growth, passion, fertility and beauty.

Ylang-ylang: Ylang-ylang symbolises sensuality and emotional healing, nourishes the heart and can work to heal deep emotional trauma.

Jasmine: Jasmine attracts love – romantic, spiritual and unconditional. It also supports purification, healing and self-confidence. Jasmine is associated with the moon, supporting women's cycles.

Sweet orange: Sweet orange is commonly used for acceptance and focus. It's known for its powers to uplift mood and promote healing.

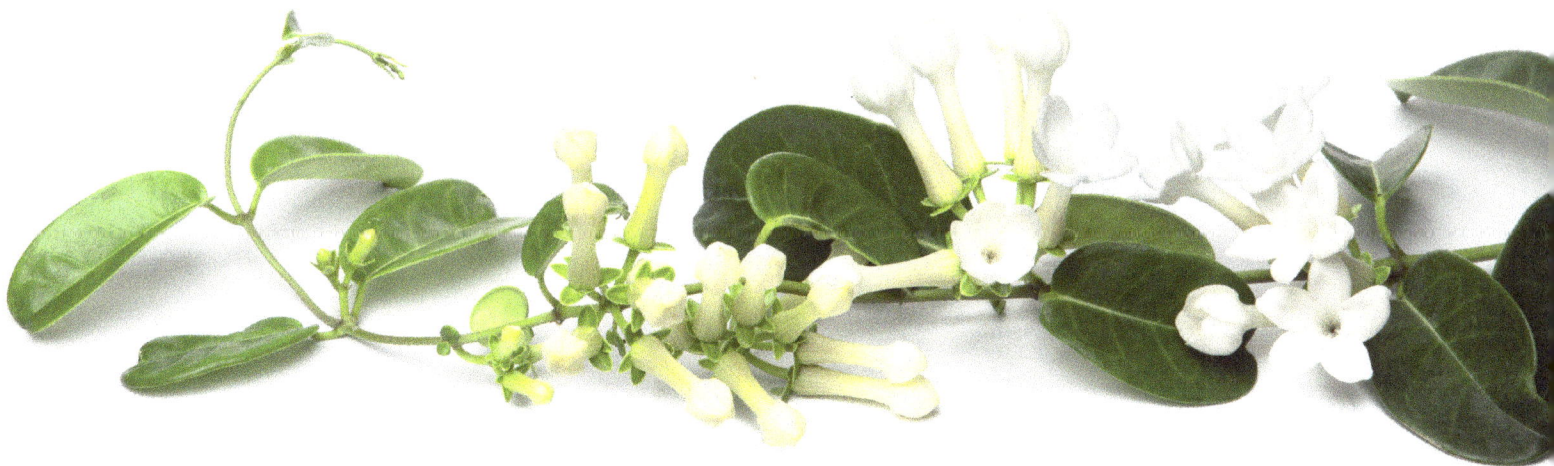

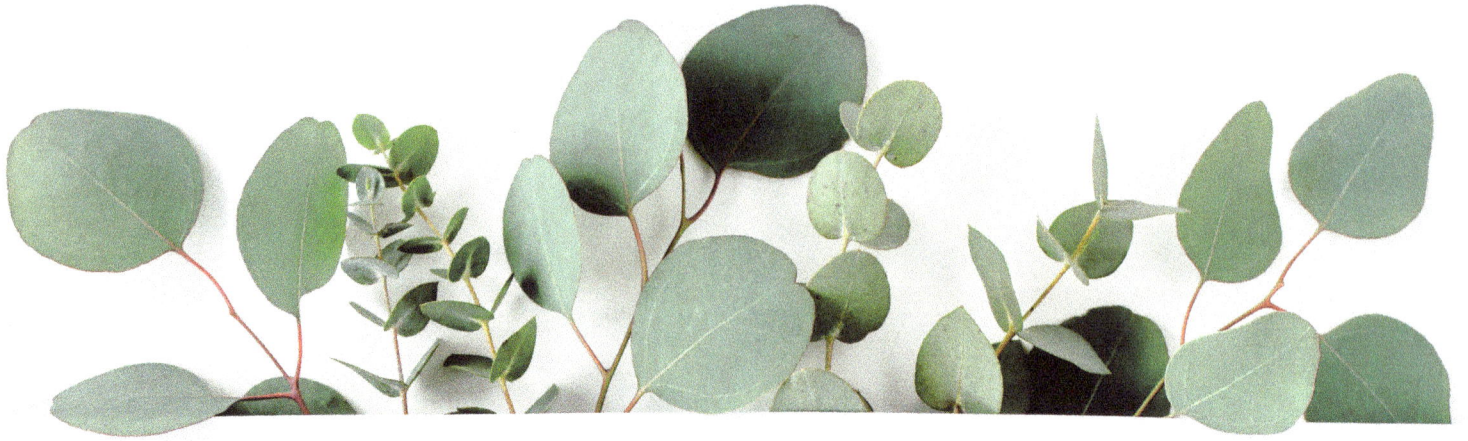

The light in you needs to
shine brighter than
the light on you.

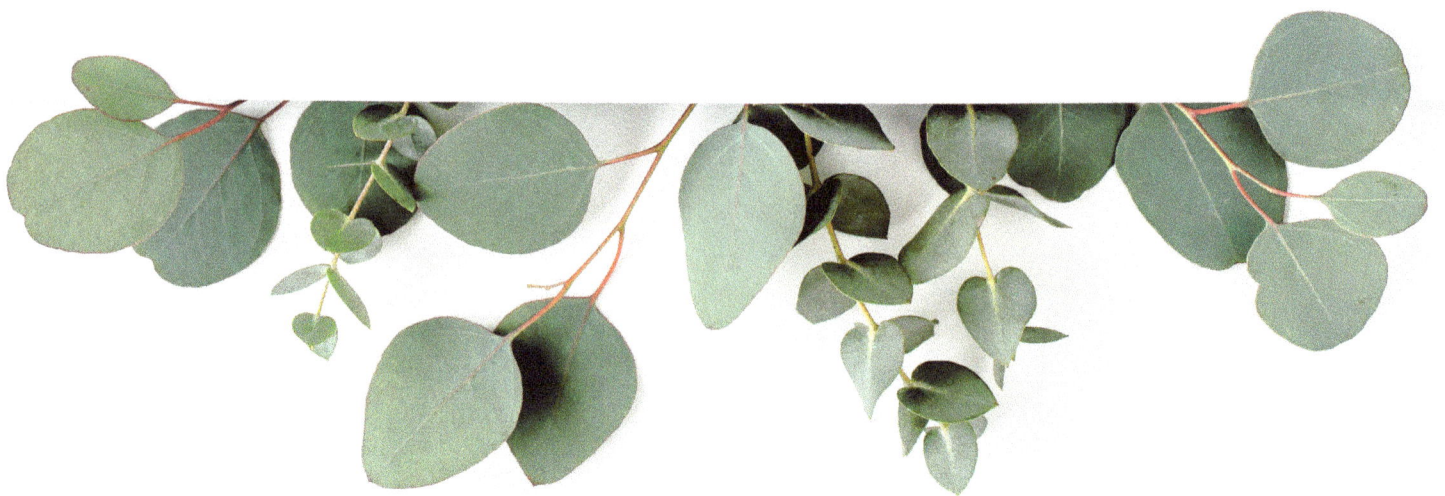

Amethyst / Cleanse

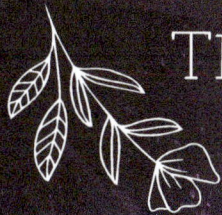

The essence of love, purification, and divine connection.

The Amethyst roll-on is a blend of Grapefruit, Lemon, Bergamot, Cardamom, and Sage.

You can apply the oil to your pulse points. The roller bottle also contains Amethyst crystals to enhance and energise the crown chakra and the essential oils.

DISCOVER THIS
PRODUCT

INGREDIENTS

Gemstone
Amethyst

Pure essential oils

Grapefruit: Grapefruit cleanses aura and mental body and clears mental chatter.

Lemon: Lemon signifies balance and strength and awakens the third eye.

Bergamot: Bergamot relieves stress, grief, depression and stability.

Cardamom: Cardamom symbolises love, sensuality, spiritual awakening, insight and wisdom.

Sage: Sage is the herb of protection, clearing, purification and ritual.

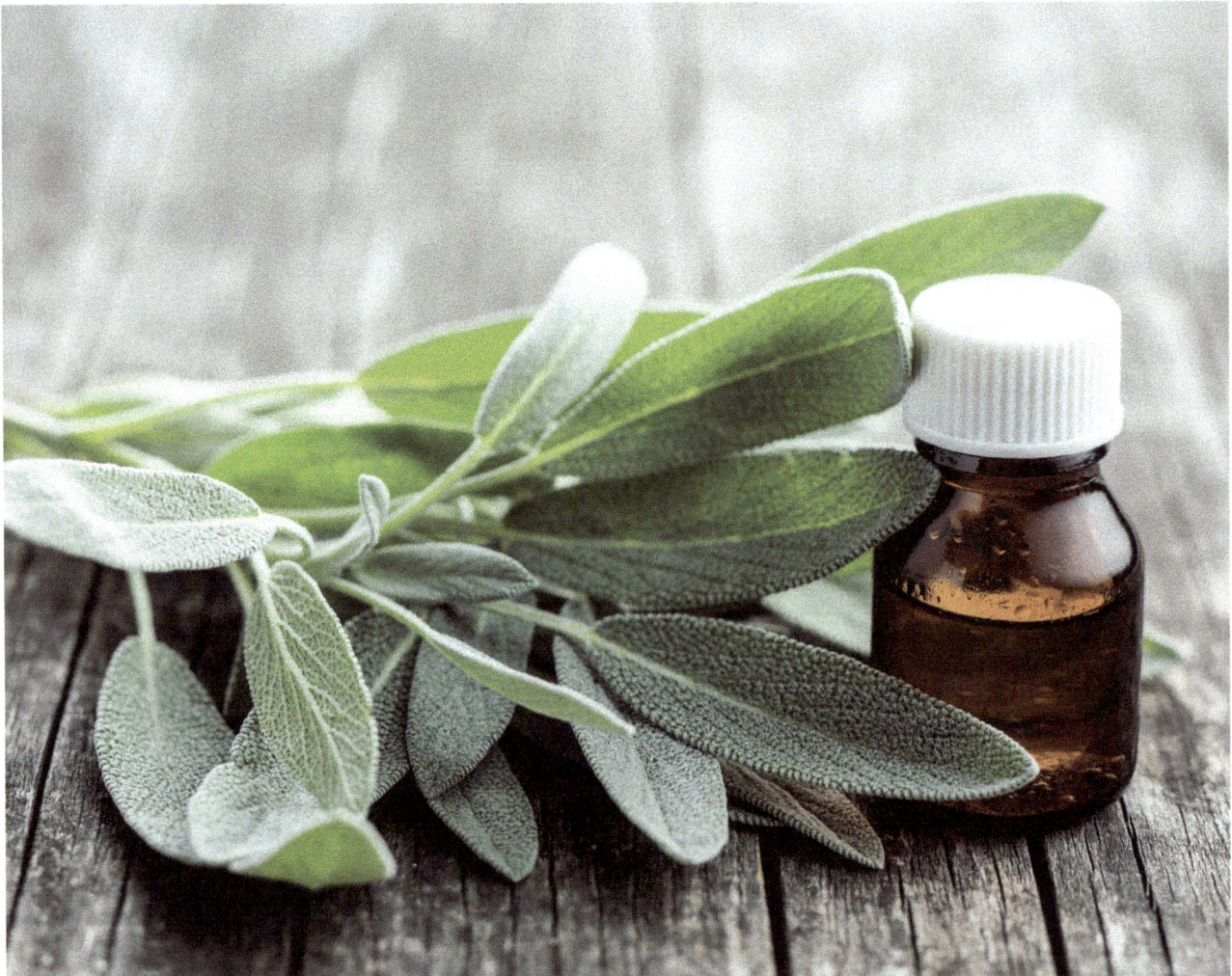

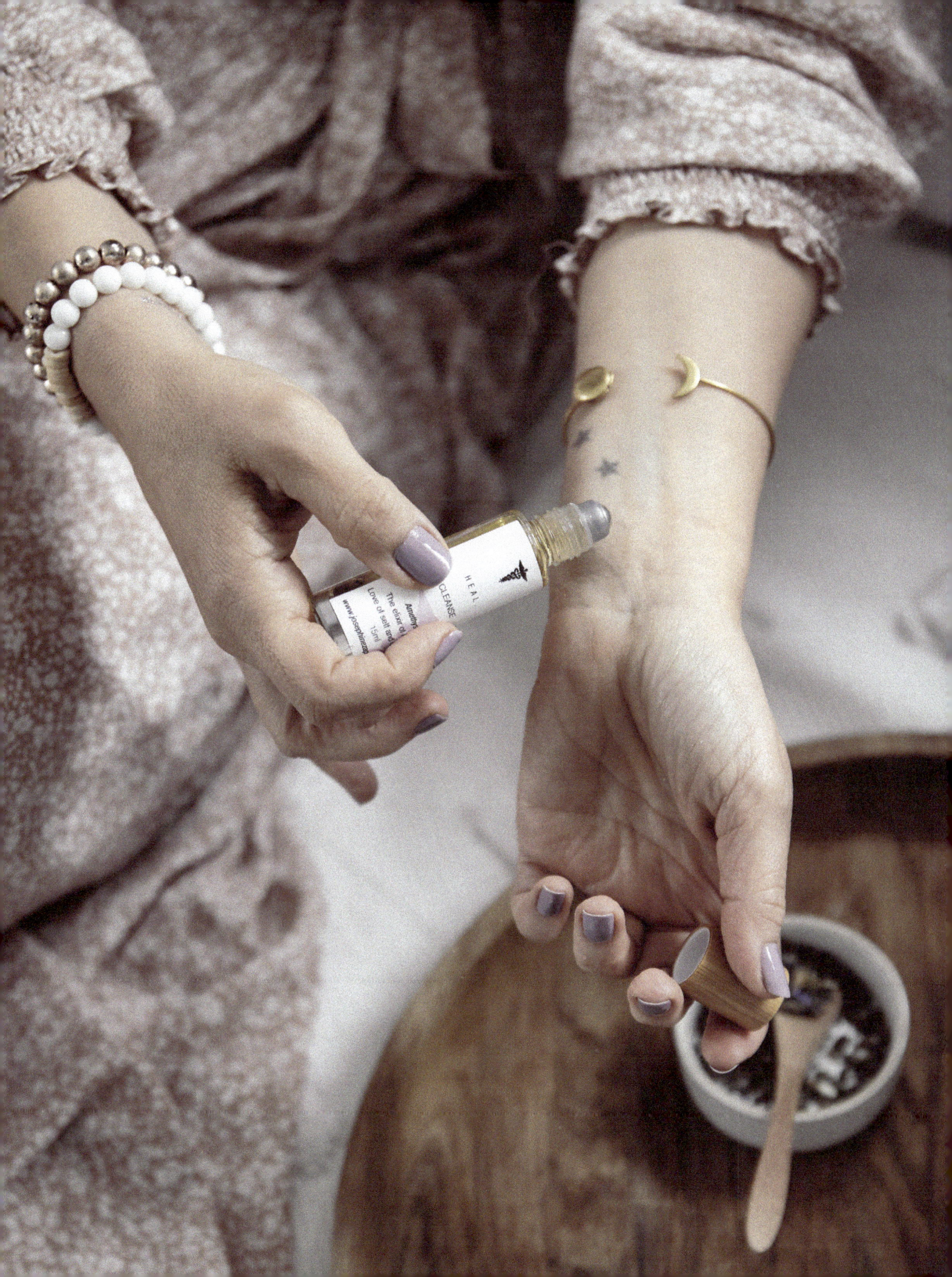

Pearl / Protection

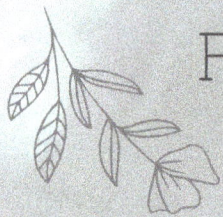

Feminine powers of wisdom, nurturing, and intuition. Powers of the mystical moon and purification.

The Pearl roll-on is a blend of Lavender, Ylang-ylang, Frankincense, Cedarwood atlas, and Sandalwood, with carrier oil: Camelia.

You can apply the oil to your pulse points. The roller bottle also contains the gemstone Pearl to enhance and energise the third eye chakra and the essential oils.

INGREDIENTS

Gemstone
Pearl

DISCOVER THIS
PRODUCT

Pure essential oils

Lavender: Lavender is responsible for cleansing the mind, body and spirit; it eases stress and anxiety and encourages purity and devotion. It also resonates with the crown chakra and connection to the higher mind.

Ylang-ylang: Ylang-ylang symbolises sensuality and emotional healing. It nourishes the heart and aids in healing deep emotional trauma.

Frankincense: Frankincense is healing and soothing; it lifts the vibration in the body, and purifies and releases inflammation.

Cedarwood atlas: Cedarwood atlas is extremely grounding and balancing and supports meditative states of consciousness.

Sandalwood: Sandalwood is cleansing and calming with a high vibrational frequency, which makes it a powerful aid in supporting manifestation and all creative endeavours.

Carrier oil: Camelia.

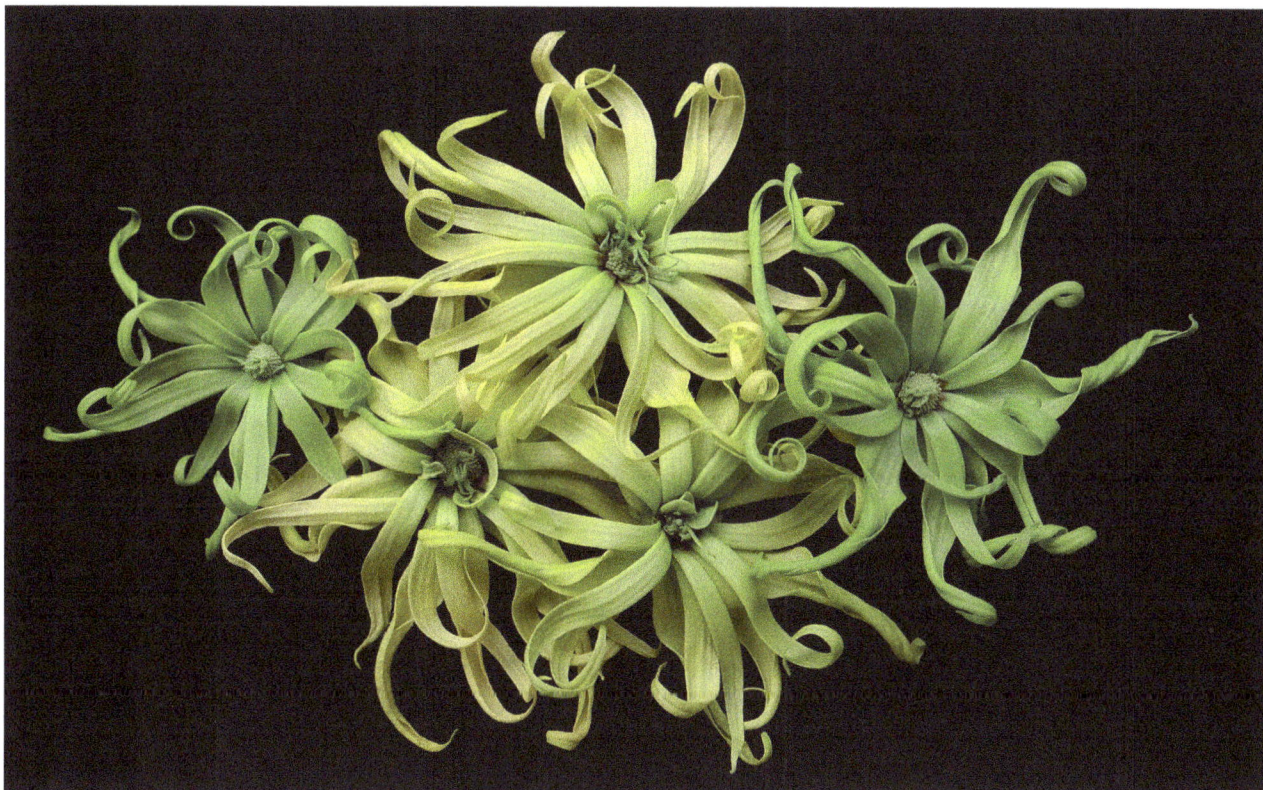

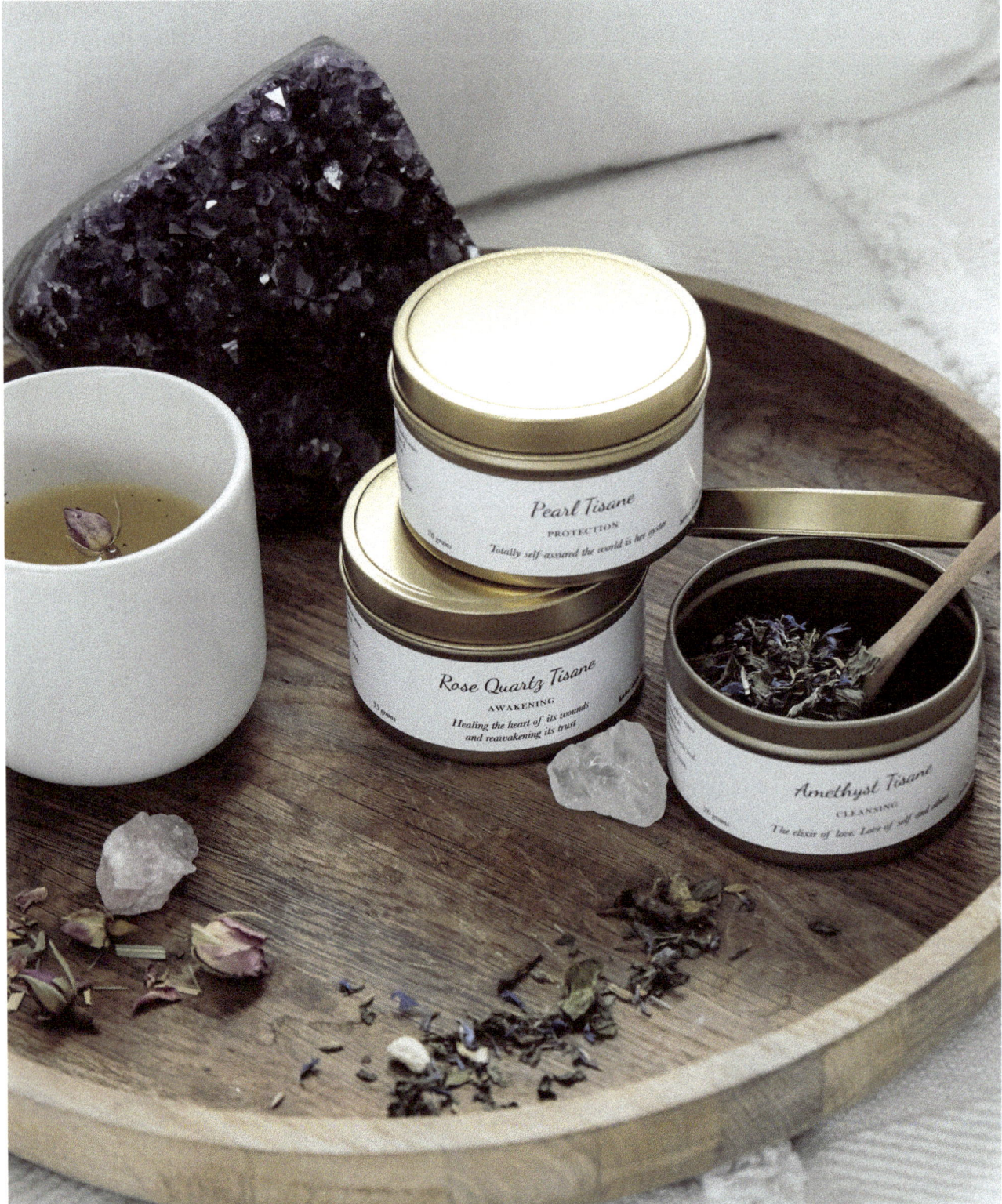

HERBAL TEAS

The Experience

HEAL. teas are caffeine-free herbal infusions.

HEAL. signature herbal blends are a unique combination of natural ingredients, traditionally used in herbal medicine to purify, calm and support natural healing and intent.

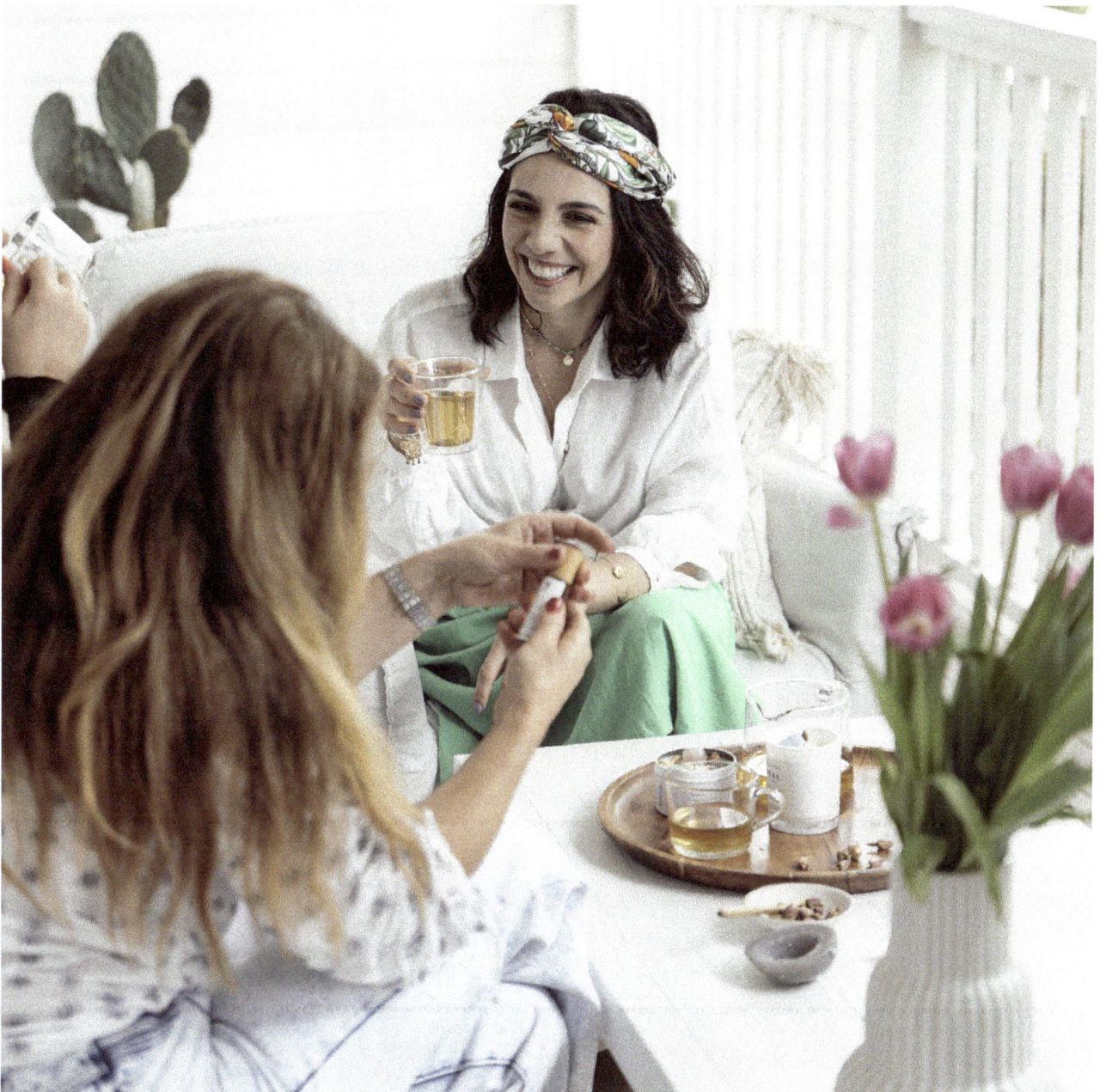

The healing benefits of herbs are extraordinary, and here are some of my personal favourites not yet in the HEAL. range. I love their taste, aroma, and beneficial therapeutic value.

Calendula
Botanical Name: *Calendula officinalis*

Drink it, steam it or soak in it. ♣ Calendula is traditionally used for postpartum recovery and wounds that do not heal properly. It has anti-inflammatory, antibacterial, and antimicrobial activity. Indicated use for sore throats, menstrual cramps, teeth, or gum irritations. Calendula can be incorporated into women's healthcare healing practises such as the abundant tradition of yoni steaming used in many cultures around the world for libido support and vulval/vaginal circulation.

Hibiscus
Botanical Name: *Hibiscus sabdariffa*

Traditionally known to help reduce blood pressure, body weight and appetite, and hold anti-diabetic qualities. Hibiscus is rich in vitamin C and antioxidants and can also be incorporated into women's healthcare healing and reconnection practices for reproductive organs.

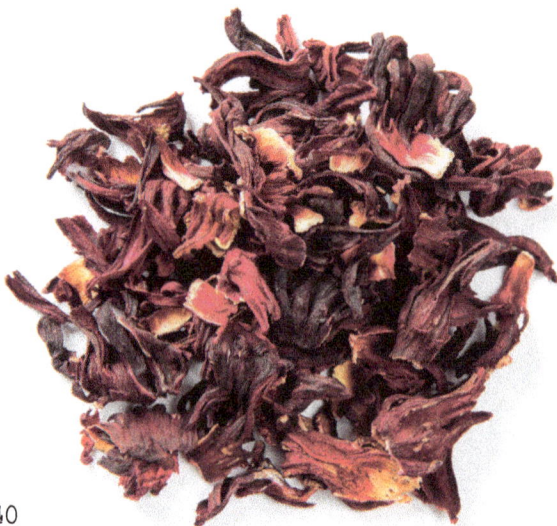

Shatavari
Botanical name: *Asparagus racemosus*

Traditionally known for its aphrodisiac, antidepressant, and anti-anxiety benefits, this herb can increase fertility and help balance and support reproductive organs. Can also be used as a diuretic, relieve bloating and menstrual cramps

Saffron
Botanical name: *Crocus sativus*

Traditionally known as an aphrodisiac and antidepressant, saffron can help balance menstruation, hormones, and skin. Saffron's homeopathic preparation is indicated for dark and copious menses, and the mental symptoms of sudden changes from happy to melancholy. Often prescribed for acquiring 'a happy heart'. Chinese medicine calls it the 'queen of herbs' for its extremely powerful boost in women's libido.

Black Cohosh
Botanical name: *Actaea racemosa* or *Cimicifuga racemosa*

Traditionally used in herbal medicine for the management of polycystic ovaries (PCOS) and associated oligo/amenorrhoea. Also known to be useful for menopausal symptoms, as a sedative for anxiety, and reducing the size of uterine fibroids in menopausal women. The homeopathic substance *cimicifuga racemosa* is indicated for amenorrhoea and dark, profuse menses.

"Looking deeply into your tea, you see that you are drinking fragrant plants that are the gift of Mother Earth."

– Thich Nhat Hanh

Tea is a universal drink, it's the second most popular drink in the world, after water. The healing qualities of sipping tea has been proven in many different cultures, all over the world, for thousands of years. It's part of our combined heritage, connection, and rituals.

Herbal teas in particular offer many health benefits and each have their own qualities and medicinal properties. They're also considered part of our daily H_2O hydration intake and nourishment.

The current HEAL. range includes herbal ingredients that were selected carefully because they aligned with my vision for the three signature blends: Rose Quartz, Amethyst, and Pearl. The ingredients match the experience of each blend. For Rose Quartz, the experience is: *Awakening. Healing the heart of its wounds. Love and trust.* Therefore, the ingredients I chose embody the qualities and spiritual uses of purification, awareness, and self-love. Amethyst embodies the experience of *Cleanse*, and Pearl is *Protection*, therefore their ingredients directly match the experience.

All three signature herbal blends are a unique combination of natural organic ingredients traditionally used in herbal medicine to purify, calm, and support natural healing. They are ideal for people of all walks of life and support their individual needs.

TESTIMONIALS

I have used all three of these natural herbal teas from HEAL. by Josephine and am very impressed with the thoughtful list of ingredients in each one.

I find it hard to specify my favourite as each one had a calming and relaxing effect on me.

The Amethyst Tisane helps with bowel issues e.g., constipation. The Rose Quartz Tisane has the refreshing flavour of the citrus and ginger which helped in clearing my chest.

The Pearl Tisane helps me sleep better, it's very relaxing.

I am delighted to recommend these teas which are beautifully presented.
D. Gonzalez, July 27, 2023

As a big lover of herbal tea, I absolutely got lost in the aroma, deliciousness, and therapeutic values of the teas. Amethyst eased my stomach discomfort; Pearl helps relax me when stressed, and my current favourite, Rose Quartz, is packed with beautiful combination of botanicals. I appreciate their ability to help release impurities from my body and deliver a feel-good energy.
J. Banach, July 30, 2023

I'm thrilled to share my experience with the Rose Quartz Tisane, instant pure qualities and freshness were clearly presented in my first sip. I am not usually a tea drinker, but I was pleasantly elated with the taste and serene properties it placed my system in. Perfect in the evening as it's very calming and relaxing as I wind down for bed. Truly a 5-star product.
C. Lewis, August 5, 2023

Rose Quartz / Awakening

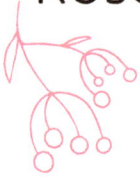

Organic ingredients: Lemongrass, Lemon myrtle leaf, Ginger root, Licorice root, Rose petal.

INGREDIENTS

Lemongrass
Botanical name: *Cymbopogon citratus*

Part used: Leaf

Flavour: Earthy, zesty

Traditionally used in herbal medicine for antibacterial, antimicrobial, relaxant, diaphoretic and antioxidant properties.

Indications: Lemongrass is good for respiratory conditions and gastrointestinal infections. Lemongrass can be calming to the nervous and musculoskeletal systems.

Spiritual uses: Lemongrass heightens awareness and purifies the mind. It can help us let go of the past.

Lemon myrtle
Botanical name: *Backhousia citriodora*

Part used: Leaf

Flavour: Citrus, lemon

Traditionally, Lemon myrtle has been used in herbal medicine as an antiseptic and a calmative as it has a relaxing effect.

Indications: The common cold, influenza and bronchitis, as well as indigestion and other irritable gut disorders.

Spiritual uses: Lemon myrtle is used for intuitive working and clears the mind.

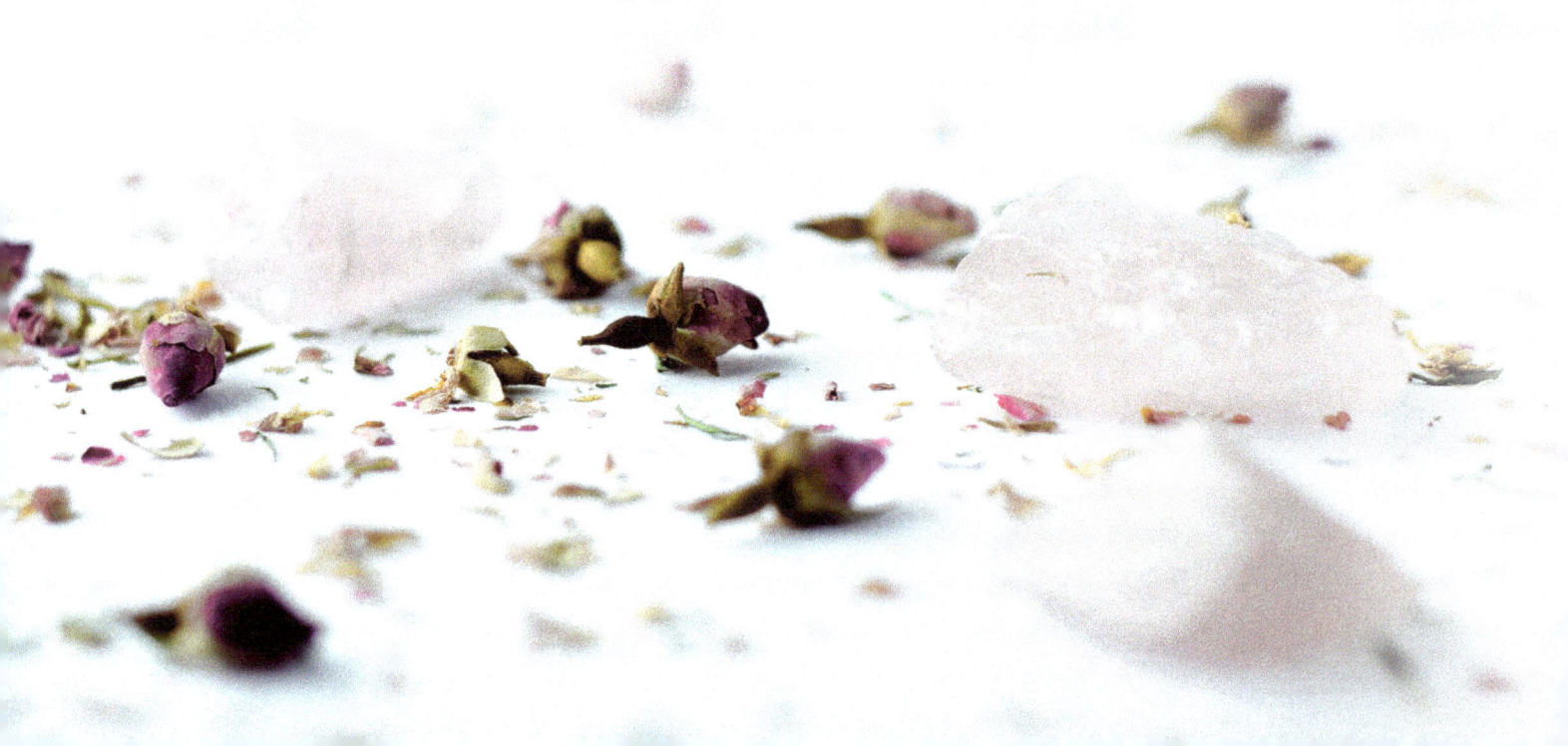

Ginger

Botanical name: *Zingiber officinale*

Part used: Root

Flavour: Pungent, spicy

Traditionally, Ginger has been used in herbal medicine as an anti-inflammatory, circulatory stimulant and antioxidant.

Indications: Nausea and vomiting associated with travel and morning sickness. It has also been used for intestinal colic, fever, arthritis, endometriosis, and migraine headaches. It can be warming for cold constitutions.

Spiritual uses: Ginger increases energy, personal power and awakens us.

Licorice

Botanical name: *Glycyrrhiza glabra*

Part used: Root

Flavour: Sweet

Traditionally used in herbal medicine as an adaptogen and adrenal restorative for stress. It also has anti-inflammatory and demulcent properties.

Indications: Respiratory conditions such as asthma, bronchitis and coughs; skin disorders such as eczema, psoriasis and acne; gastrointestinal disorders including gastritis, ulcers, irritable bowel syndrome and constipation. It is also excellent for sugar cravings.

Spiritual uses: Licorice root is used to heighten power; it is a potent fortifier of love and connection.

Rose

Botanical name: *Rosa centifolia*

Part used: Flower

Flavour: Floral

Traditionally used in herbal medicine, rose has been used to soothe the nerves and emotional and psychological state of mind.

Spiritual uses: Rose calms the nervous system and heals the heart centre. It is often used for self-compassion and self-love.

DISCOVER THIS
PRODUCT

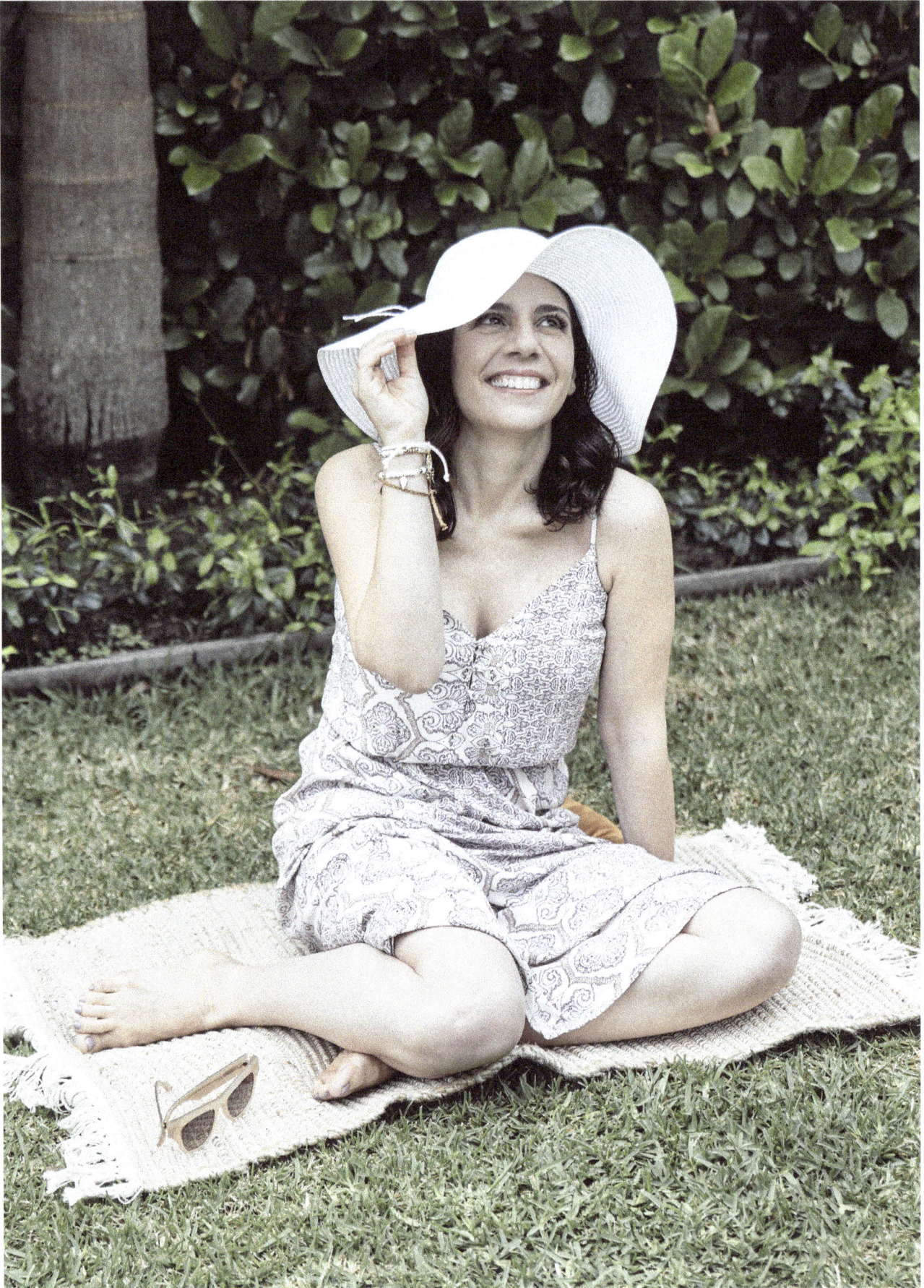

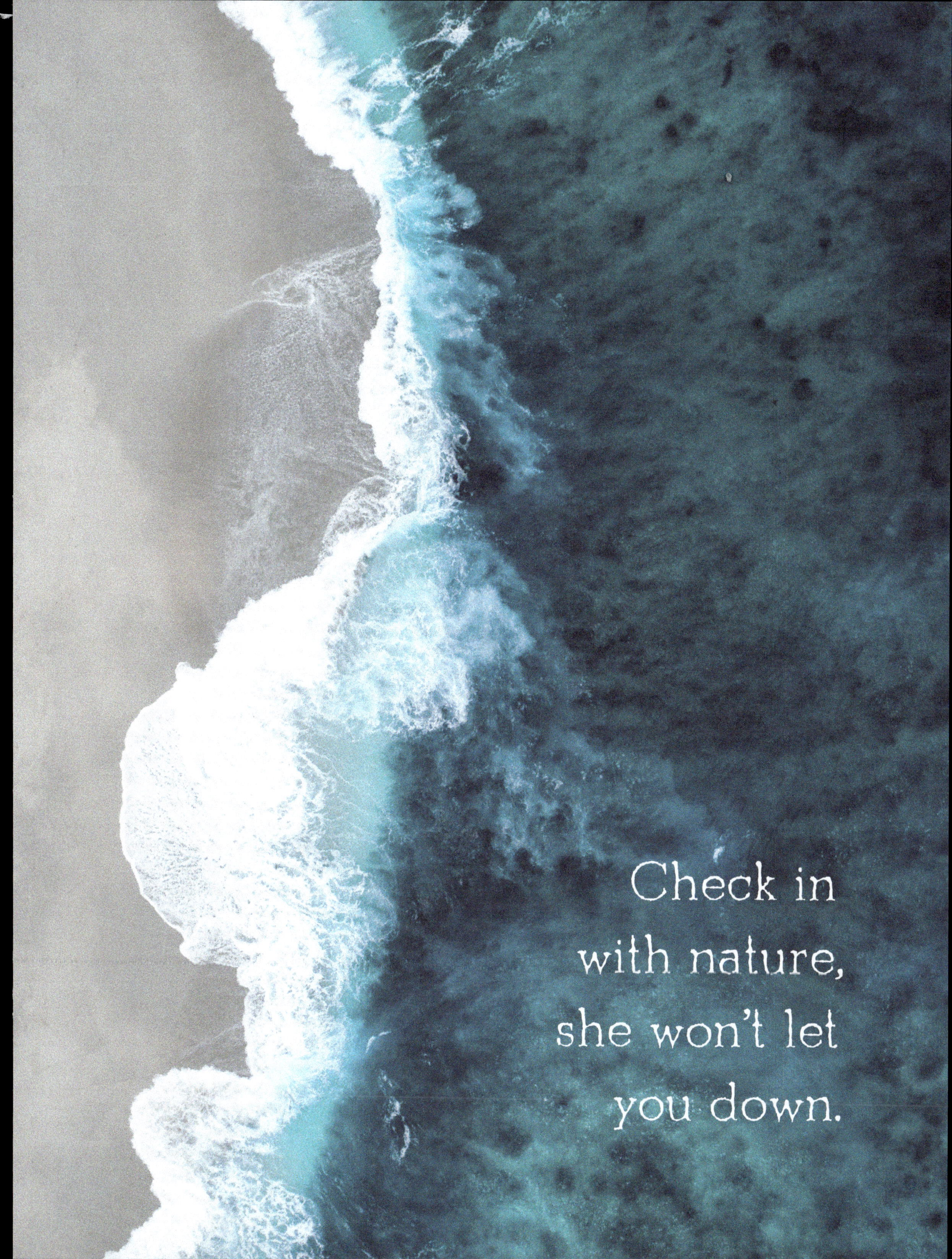

Check in
with nature,
she won't let
you down.

Amethyst / Cleanse

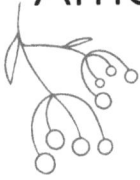

Organic ingredients: Peppermint leaf, Fennel seed, Marshmallow root, Blue cornflower, Nettle leaf.

INGREDIENTS

Marshmallow
Botanical name: *Althaea officinalis*

Part used: Root

Flavour: Sweet

Traditionally used in herbal medicine as an emollient for irritated mucous membranes of the gut and respiratory tract, it has a softening and soothing action.

Spiritual uses: Marshmallow root is comforting, soothing and protective and it supports self-love.

Fennel
Botanical name: *Foeniculum vulgare*

Part used: Seed

Flavour: Sweet, anise

Traditionally used in herbal medicine as a carminative (relieving colic and wind) and anti- inflammatory.

Indications: Bloating, wind and tummy discomfort.

Spiritual uses: Fennel is used for healing, protection, purification, strength, vitality, passion and courage.

Peppermint
Botanical name: *Mentha x piperita*

Part used: Leaf

Flavour: Menthol, cleansing, refreshing

Traditionally used in herbal medicine as an antibacterial, antiseptic, cooling and carminative (relieving wind and colic) herb. Peppermint is also a diaphoretic (promoting perspiration) and acts as a cholagogue (increasing the flow of bile).

Indications: Colds, intestinal colic, indigestion, flatulent dyspepsia, nausea and vomiting during pregnancy, and irritable bowel syndrome.

Spiritual uses: Peppermint is an uplifting, energetic plant that stimulates physical healing.

DISCOVER THIS
PRODUCT

Blue cornflower

Botanical name: *Centaurea cyanus*

Part used: Flower

Flavour: Floral

Traditionally used for its decorative purpose in tea blends and to give a slight blue tint to the steeped tea.

Spiritual uses: Blue cornflower is used to enhance psychic abilities, fertility, love, sex, and abundance.

Nettle

Botanical name: *Urtica dioica*

Part used: Leaf

Flavour: Herbal

Traditionally used in herbal medicine as a nutritive and astringent indicated for inflamed and impure skin, Nettle is also cleansing.

Spiritual uses: Nettle leaves are protective, dispelling fear, clearing energy and strengthening will.

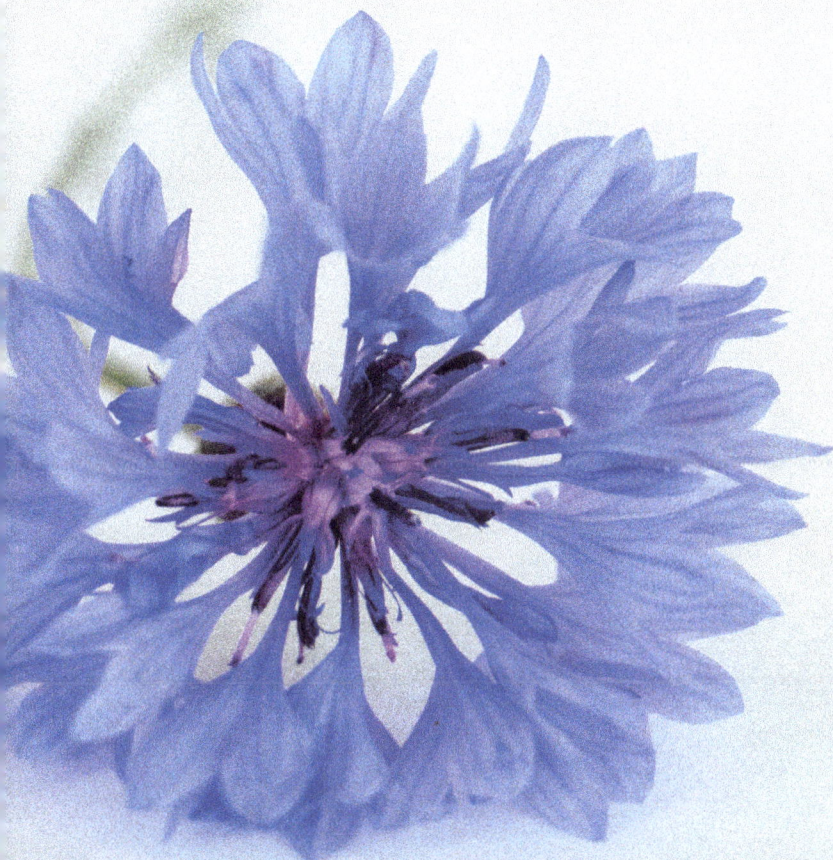

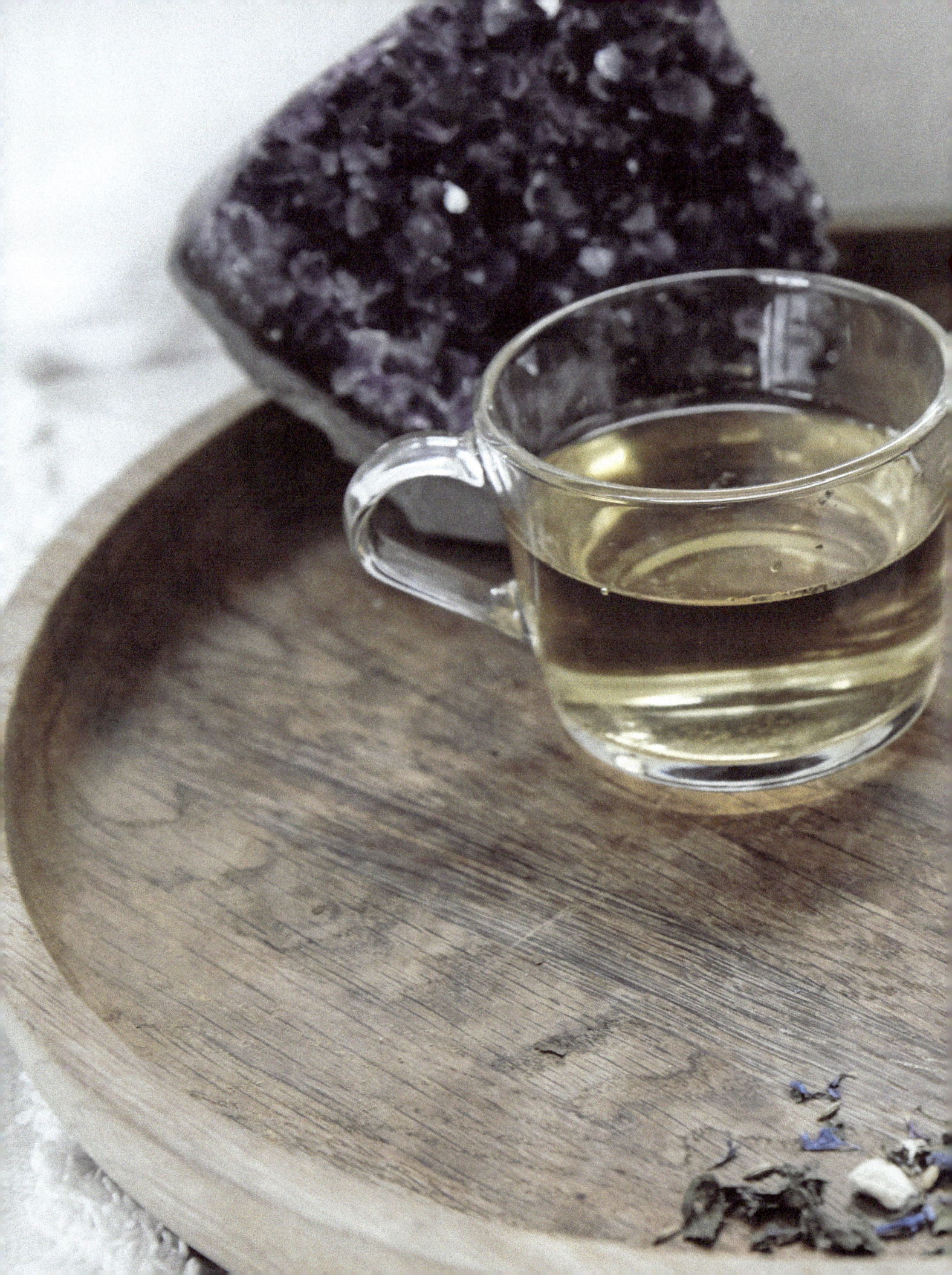

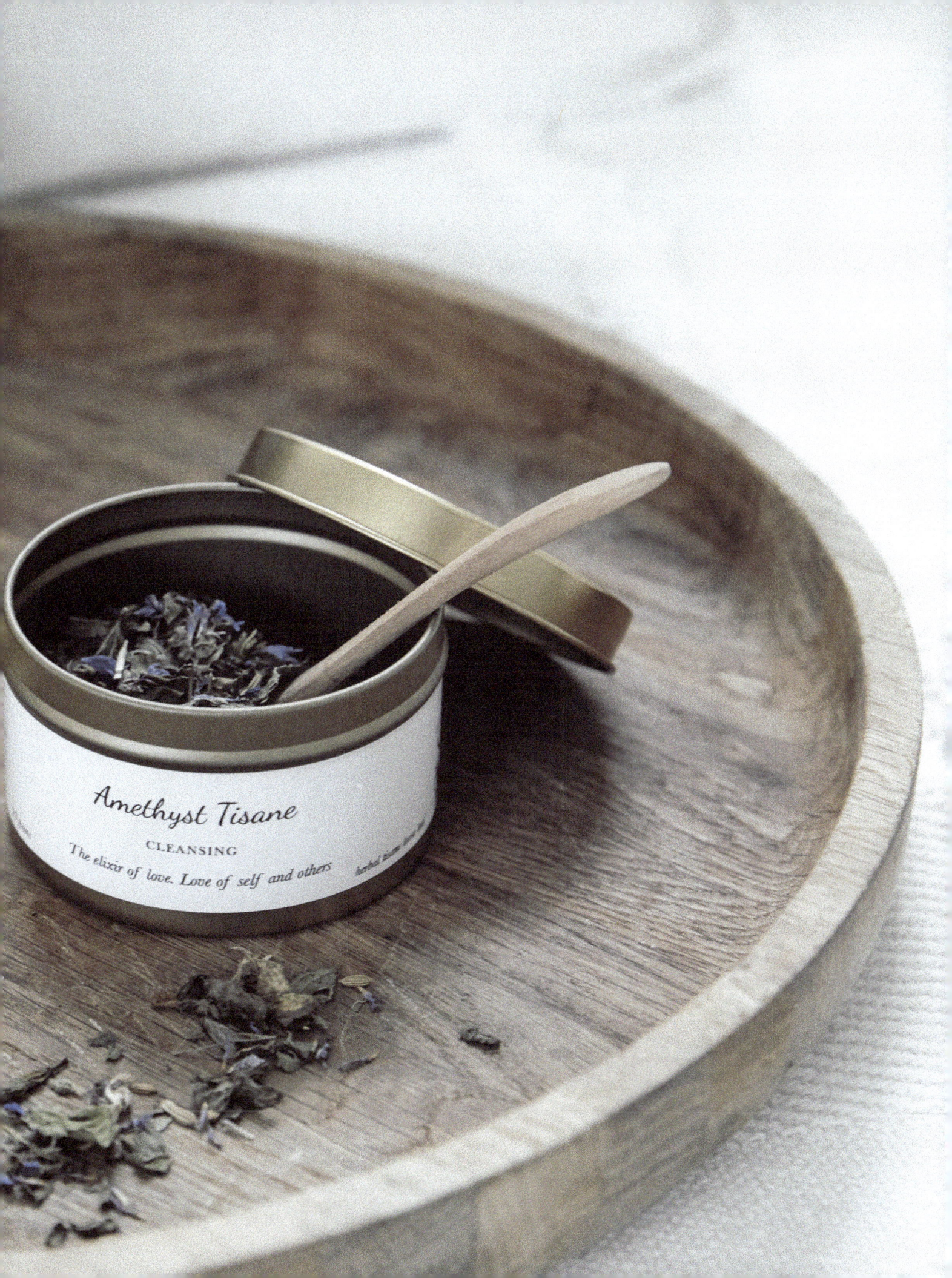

Amethyst Tisane

CLEANSING

The elixir of love. Love of self and others

herbal tisane loose leaf

Pearl / Protection

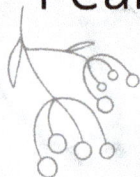

Organic ingredients: Holy basil leaf, Rosemary leaf, Lavender flower, Sage leaf.

DISCOVER THIS PRODUCT

INGREDIENTS

Holy basil
Botanical name: *Ocimum tenuiflorum*

Part used: Leaf

Flavour: Herbal

Traditionally known in herbal medicine as a plant that is considered sacred in Hinduism, Holy basil is known for its restorative and spiritual properties. It acts as an adaptogen to help regulate stress.

Spiritual uses: Holy basil nurtures the spirit, helping you to balance the chakras and find your centre.

Rosemary
Botanical name: *Salvia rosmarinus*

Part used: Leaf

Flavour: Herbal

Traditionally used in herbal medicine as an antioxidant, antimicrobial, spasmolytic (relieving spasms), carminative, mild analgesic, and circulatory stimulant. Rosemary is used to support healing for headaches, anxiety, depression, poor concentration and memory, improvement of hepatic and biliary function (supporting fat digestion).

Spiritual uses: Rosemary is used for protection and cleansing, but also for love, healing and feminine power.

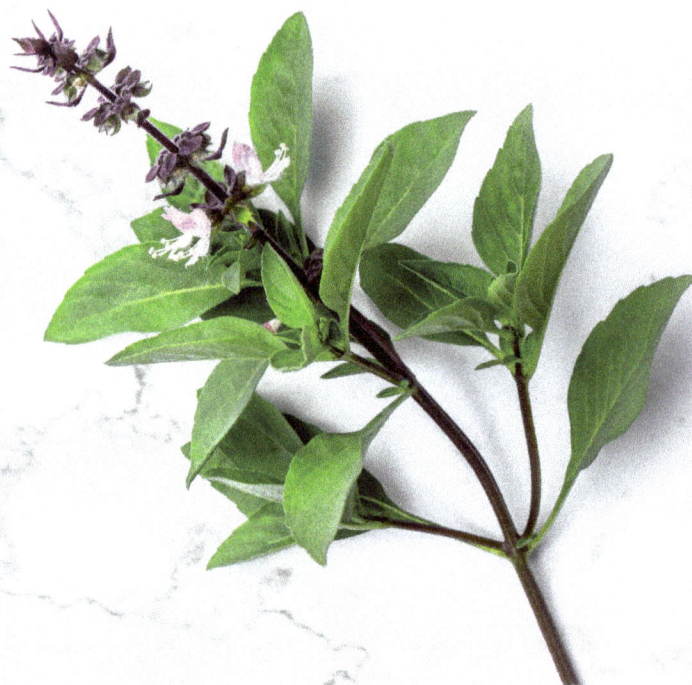

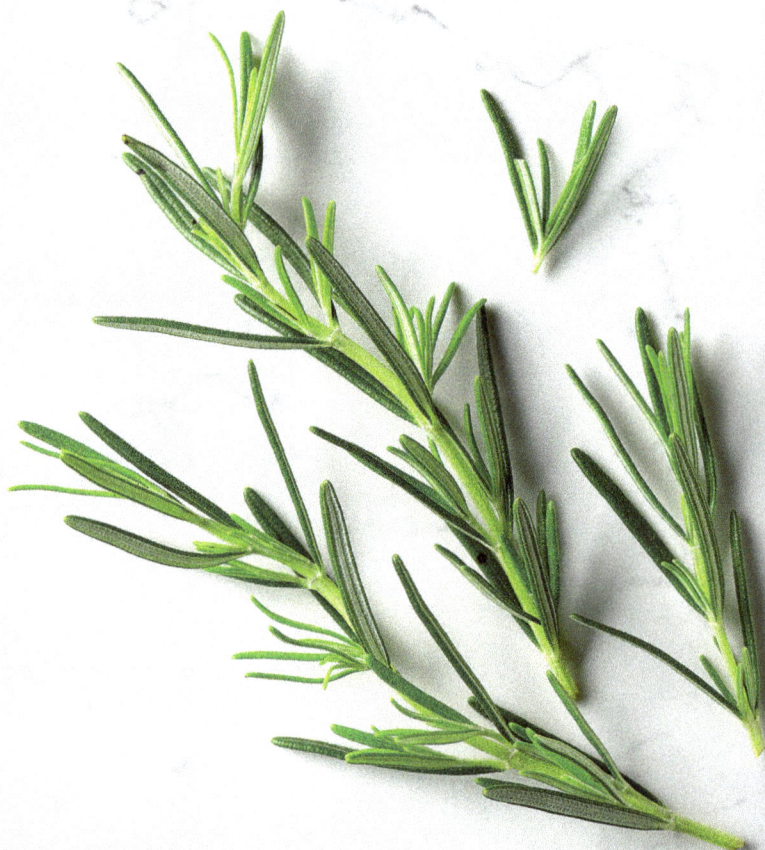

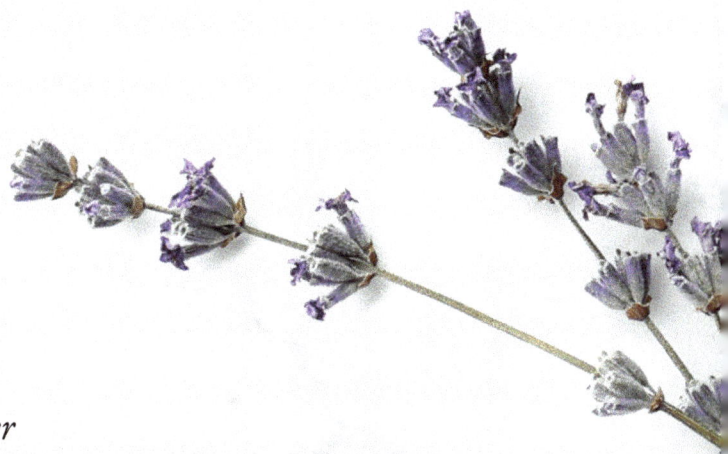

Lavender

Botanical name: *Lavender angustifolia*

Part Used: Flower

Flavour: Floral

Lavender has traditionally been used in herbal medicine as an antidepressant, carminative (relieving colic and wind), and muscle and nerve relaxant. It helps relieve muscle spasms and aids relaxation during times of stress or anxiety, and can be used to unwind before sleep.

Indications: Intestinal colic or digestive weakness, flatulent dyspepsia, headache, and menopausal symptoms.

Spiritual uses: Lavender is soothing and relaxing, can cleanse the house of negative energy and is used as a beacon of love.

Sage

Botanical name: *Salvia officinalis*

Part used: Leaf

Flavour: Herbal

Traditionally used in herbal medicine as an antiseptic and anhidrotic (reducing perspiration), this herb has been traditionally used during menopause and for the treatment of excess perspiration and hot flushes.

Spiritual uses: Sage has strong cleansing and purifying properties and helps clear out negative energy.

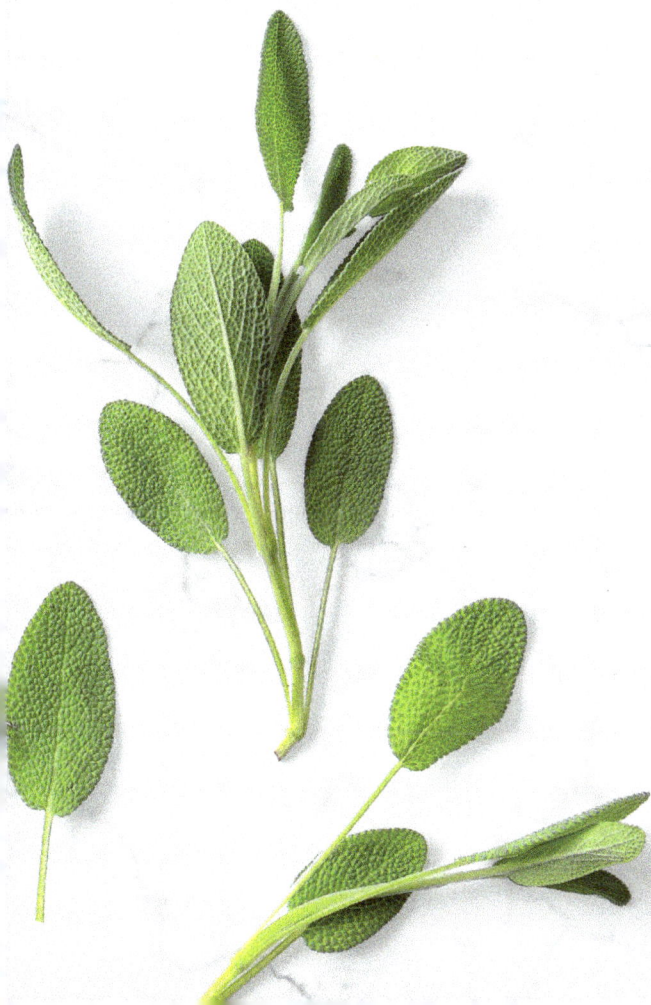

HOMEOPATHIC REMEDIES

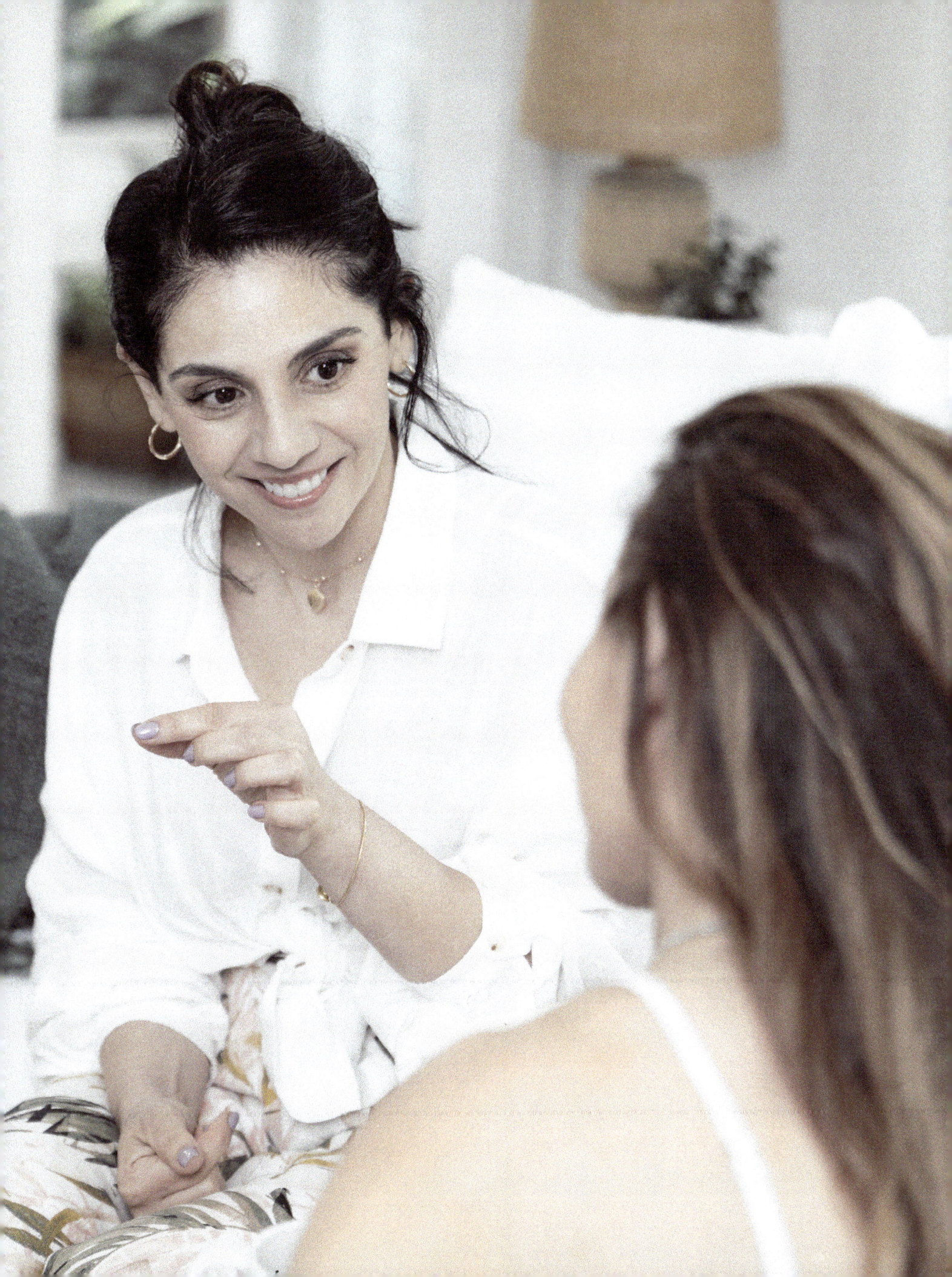

About homeopathy

Most chronic conditions are multifactorial. Homeopathy will address the psychosomatic, genetic, and miasmatic causes, but it is not a substitute for solving nutritional deficiency.

I often tell patients that after treatment, they may feel very different. The way you respond to things is going to change first, and when you sustain that, the symptoms you are experiencing fall away; they no longer need to be there to teach or show you what you need to learn, as you now know it.

On some level the symptoms are revealing something, and in some instances, we can become attached to them and their purpose in our life. To love them, accept them, and then let them go can be confronting. Homeopathy works with the flow of life, because by working with the principles of nature, we allow this flow.

When we dismiss our symptoms and don't seek the root cause, we dismiss our emotions and our own inner guidance.

By allowing homeopathy to gently shift the lens through which we operate, we allow our bodies to work towards equilibrium and gently let go of what no longer serves our highest good.

Homeopathy is also useful for everyday complaints. In many first aid books available today, the art of homeopathic prescribing is oversimplified, which gives a false impression that prescribing a homeopathic remedy is simply a matter of looking up the complaint. However, this will result in the remedy working for only a percentage of those people who take it.

The tools used for prescribing are:

✦ William Boericke's *Materia Medica*, which is a full account of all the homeopathic remedies.

Fighting Weakens; Love Empowers.

✦ Dr N. M. Choudari's *A Study on Materia Medica and Repertory*, which is a cross-referenced index of the information presented in the *Materia Medica*.

In order to effectively and safely use homeopathy, an understanding of the laws and principles is essential.

Classical homeopathy is very different in approach from orthodox medicine. When you go to the doctor for an illness or other malady, you may receive treatment for the symptoms and not the root cause. However, the symptoms are there for a reason and if the reason still exists, then the problem will return, either in the same form or through a different disease or problem, as the root of the problem wasn't dealt with. The body will always find another valve in which to express the discord through. Suppressing the symptoms will only bring short-term relief.

Homeopathy has a clear understanding of the difference between suppression and real healing. With healing, the root of the problem is dealt with first, and as a result the symptoms are no longer needed and fade away.

During a consultation, the homeopath examines every aspect of the patient's life and doesn't just focus on isolated symptoms. The same patient who comes in complaining of headaches may also have depression, insecurities, low energy and a long list of other problems. A single homeopathic remedy that considers the entire picture is prescribed – this is known as constitutional prescribing.

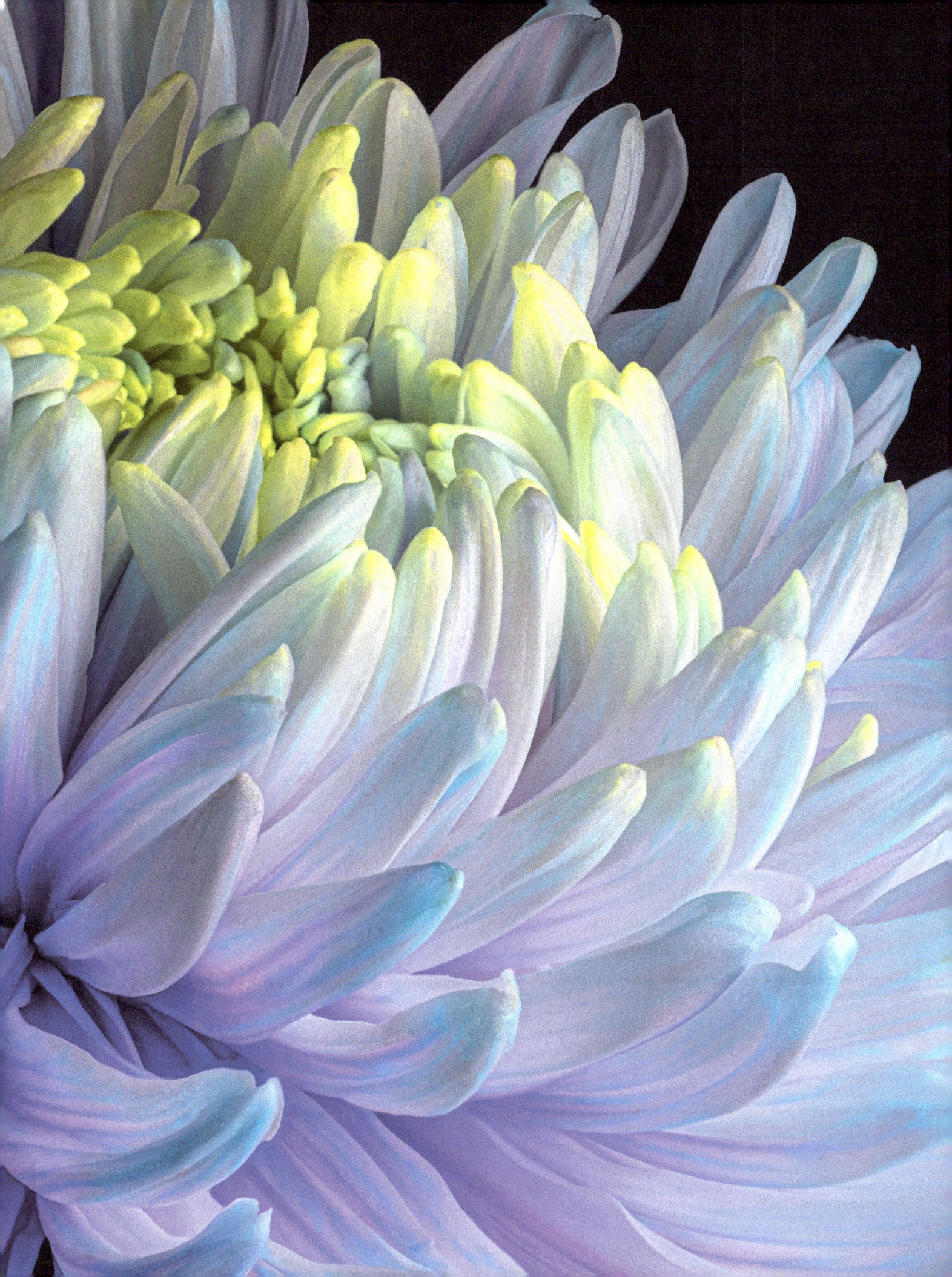

People who have had homeopathic treatment generally find that their overall state of health and wellbeing has improved. Holistic medicine, with its philosophies of health maintenance and disease treatment, is really the ordinary, commonsense medicine which has been practised for centuries. It combines the knowledge of natural sciences with experience and common sense. Natural law is based on the principles of nature, which are permanent and irrefutable and have remained unchanged since their discovery.

It is only by making choices about all of these factors that we can enjoy health to its fullest extent.

Medicines

Homeopathic medicines are a gentle way of stimulating the body's own natural response to healing.

They are sourced from nature's kingdoms – animals, plants, minerals, and diseased tissue (termed nosodes) – and are prepared by a process of step-by-step repeated dilution and succussion (vigorous hitting against a hard elastic body).

The crude substance is diluted of its toxic effects, and then succussed. The succussion is what raises its energy, and thus makes them capable of stimulating the body's own defence system and allowing it to heal itself by mimicking the diseases they aim to treat.

Correctly administered homeopathic medicines are not intrinsically dangerous. It is the body's vital force (energy flow) which is influenced, rather than its chemical balance (as in orthodox medicine). These remedies are non-habit-forming and without side effects. Homeopathy can often help patients with a multitude of ailments and is also effective in the treatment of stress, grief and depression.

What does homeopathy mean?

Homeopathy means 'similar to the suffering'. It originates from the Greek language, with *homoios* meaning similar or like and *patheia* meaning feeling or suffering. This is sometimes taken to mean 'like cures like'.

"In other words, a substance produces symptoms of illness in a well person when administered in large doses. If we administer the same substance in minute quantities, it will cure the disease in a sick person." When the substance is administered in homeopathic form, it is in minute quantities because it has been diluted then succussed.

Ecology: The opposite force to your force of desire

(Environmental science. Life science.)
Once the ecology is depressurised, and it is safe to achieve and maintain what you want, the obstacles and disease state (which is a part of the whole pull) spontaneously dissolve. *It's okay to get what you want. Appreciate the present state. Respect both parts of you.*

APHORISM 1

"The physician's high and only mission is to restore the sick to health; to cure, as it is termed."
– Samuel Hahnemann

The foremost merit of homeopathy is that while curing one disease, it does not create another.

APHORISM 2

"The highest ideal of cure is rapid, gentle, and permanent restoration of the health, or removal and annihilation of the disease in its whole extent, in the shortest, most reliable and most harmless way, on easily comprehensible principles."
– Samuel Hahnemann

The second merit of homeopathy is that the potentised drugs stimulate the power of resistance of the sick person, to destroy the diseases naturally, thus producing cure in the most natural way.

THE SIMILLIMUM

The simillimum is the remedy most indicated to the patient's presenting diseased state, and thus is most likely to restore health. When given to a healthy person, it will produce the symptoms most similar to those of the patient.

ENERGY ALIGNMENT

Align your body, realise your potential.

The next-level version of your life requires the next-level version of you. A homeopath will match the energy of the patient to the remedy, so that patients can get to the desired level of alignment.

Tabula Rasa (clean slate)

The answers are never *outside* of you.

As the potencies of your remedy increase, the *awareness* sinks deeper and deeper, and hence the realisation of your patterns.

You have all the answers. I am facilitating in deepening that *healing;* with or without a remedy.

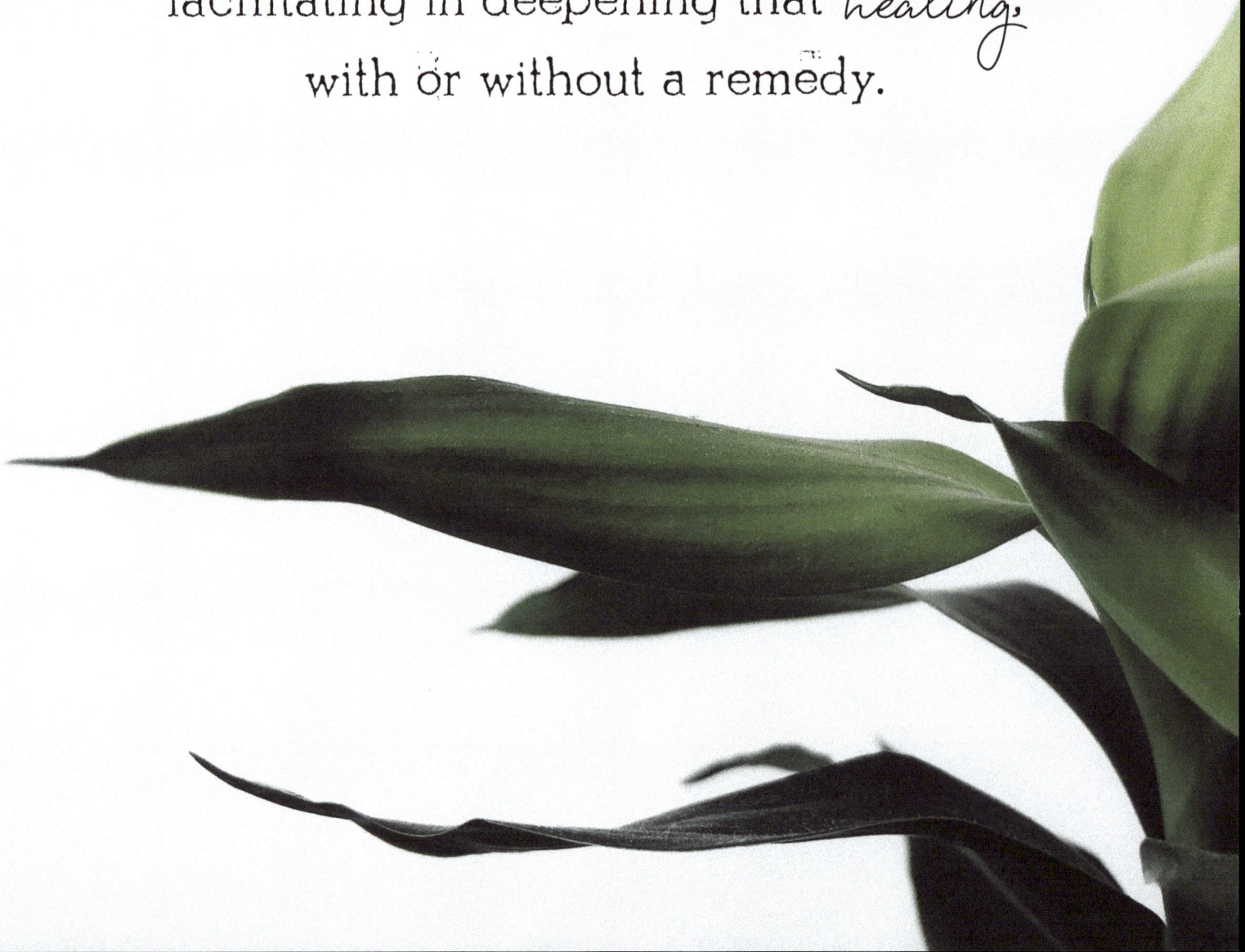

Psychosomatic, genetic and miasm factors of conditions

Most chronic conditions are multifactorial. I don't believe there's one single modality for every one person at every stage of their lives. All modalities under the complementary and alternative medicine (CAM) umbrella hold relevance as holistic healing is an integrative treatment.

Transforming the way we practise medicine, homeopathic medicines are very deep-acting and will address the psychosomatic, genetic, and miasmatic causes. They are not, however, a fix for poor nutrition, incongruous lifestyle, environmental, familial or culturally inapt circumstances.

Psychosomatic: refers to the interconnection between psyche, mind, and soma (body).

Genetic: family history; inherited genes that predispose to a specific condition.

Miasm: hereditary predisposition (deeper than a genetic cause). A miasm can include genetic predispositions to disease, but it refers to much more than a specific disease condition. The inherited miasmatic picture is expressed through the specific genetic condition and could be any of the fundamental miasms requiring treatment.

The psychology of injuries

Mind and body always speak the same language. This means that a patient who is so oversensitive physically is also going to be oversensitive and reactive mentally. This can also be expressed as overly anxious and stressed.

There are distinct types of guilt or fears that attract certain types of accidents. This is known as the psychology of injuries - such an interesting topic! - and is directly associated with the psychology of chronic disease patterns resulting from injuries that occurred years before with a common psychosomatic origin.

Example ~ While the muscle damage remedy *Arnica Montana* is given for injuries, a homeopath will also prescribe *Arnica* for the mental symptoms of guilt. This clears the mindset or attitude, and the injuries stop happening.

Calendula Officinalis (Marigold)

Pot marigold (*Calendula officinalis*) can be used for wound healing. For wounds that do not heal properly, calendula can stimulate anti-inflammatory and antimicrobial activity and antibacterial healing, as well as having an antioxidant effect. Calendula speeds up the recovery of wounds by reducing the bacterial load.

Calendula is also used for:

♣ Sore throats.

♣ Menstrual cramps.

♣ Postpartum recovery – you can help your perineum heal with a gentle 'bonding with baby' bath soak.

♣ Teeth and/or gum irritations such as haemorrhaging (bleed excessively or becoming infected) after extraction.

Calendula tincture or cream can be used as an antiseptic dressing for simple cuts, open abrasions and lacerated wounds. It takes away local pain and promotes healthy rapid healing. This multi-purpose remedy is a pot of gold.

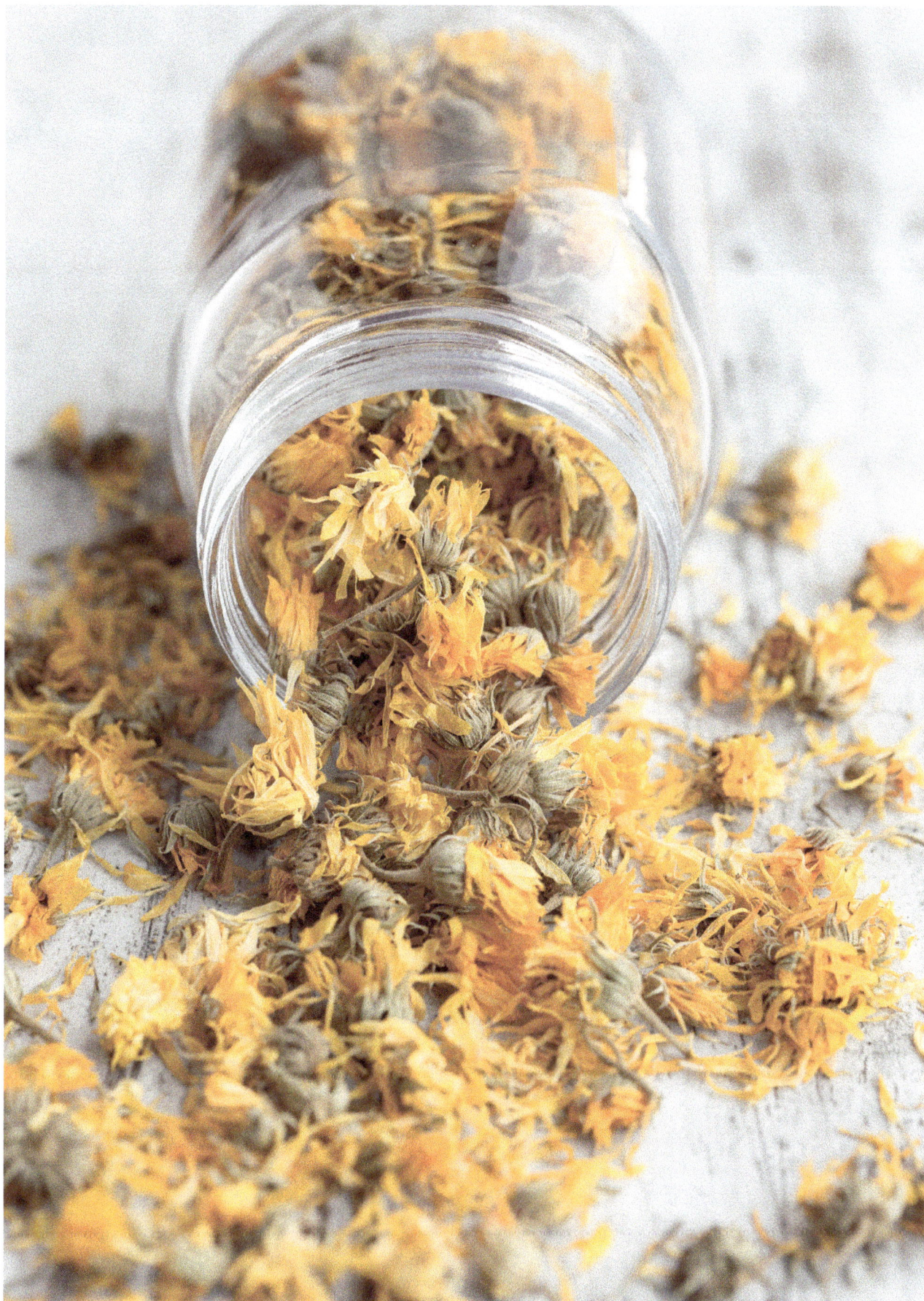

Teucrium marum (Cat thyme)

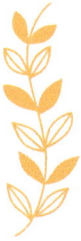

The Germander (*Lamiaceae*) family to which the teucriums belong had an important place in old herbal medicine, and homeopathy has placed similar importance on teucrium.

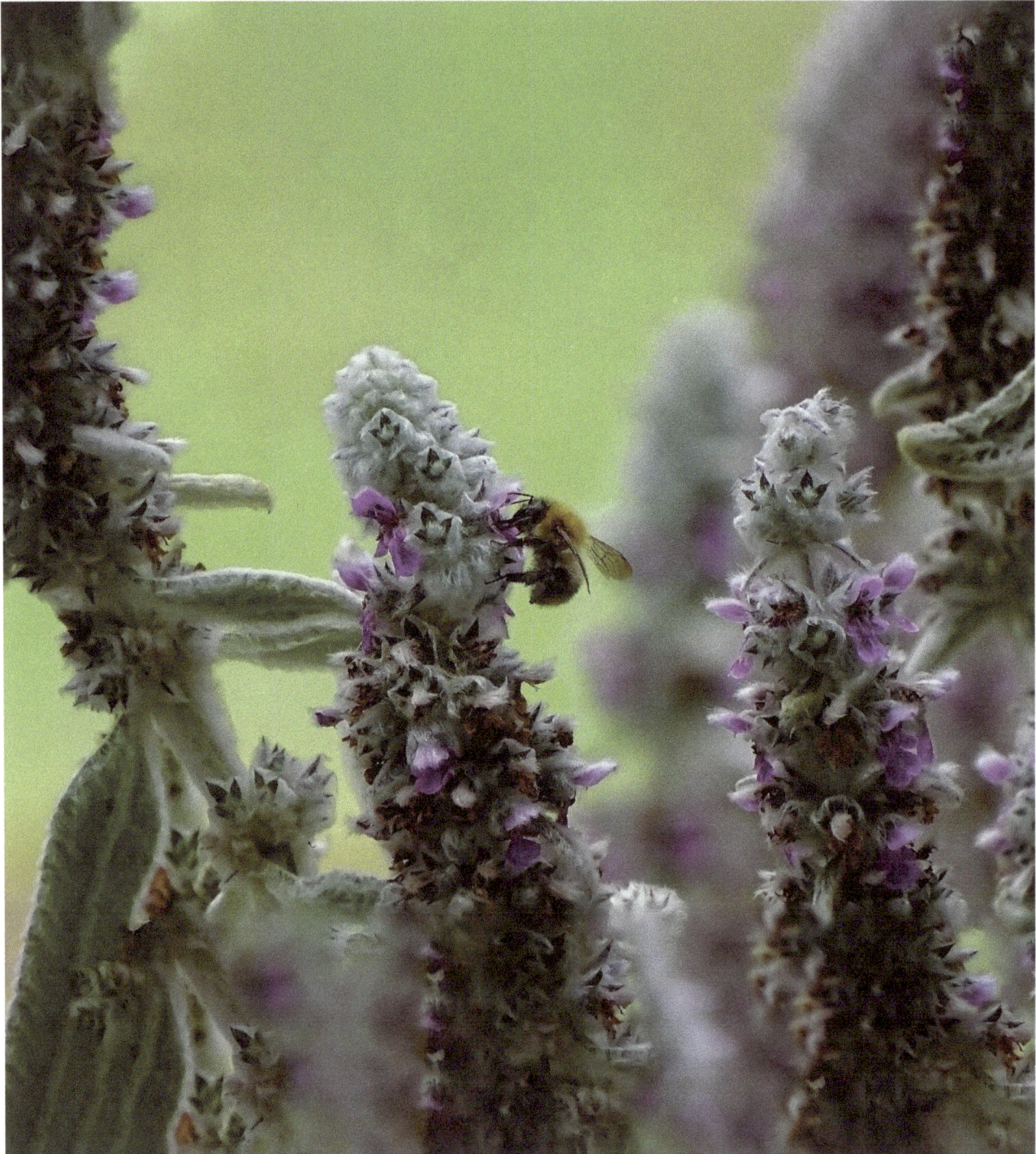

MATERIA MEDICA

The teucrium mind is a state of irritability and irascibility, with sensitiveness so great that fatigue is produced by merely hearing the conversation of others.

Nasal and rectal symptoms are common. Therefore, teucrium is the first remedy to think of when someone is experiencing chronic nasal catarrh. The nasal symptoms have led to the use of teucrium in nasal polyps.

Teucrium is suitable after too much medicine has been taken and has produced an oversensitive condition, and remedies fail to act.

Unhappy; sadness, mental depression; from becoming cold.

Weeping, crying, tearful mood (lamenting); aggravated by own weeping.

Impaired thinking; confusion; dullness of mind; sluggishness of mind; weakness of mind.

Loss of sense of smell.

Puffiness of upper eyelids. Teucrium has removed a fibrous tumour of the eyelid.

Vision blurred.

Worms. No remedy meets more threadworms than Teuc. The worms and Polypi suggest a tubercular taint, and both Teucrium MV and Teucrium Scorodonia (Wood Sage) can be used in phthisical cases.

Teuc has the craving hunger of the antipsorics and worm remedies; and it prevents sleep at night.

Nervous, irritable, sensitive.

Respiratory: there is a dry cough, tickling in trachea, mouldy taste in throat when hawking up mucous, expectoration is profuse.

Extremities: Affection of fingertips and joints of toes. Tearing pains in arms and legs. Pain of toenails as if they had grown into flesh (ingrown toenail).

Skin: Restless, Itching causes tossing about all night. Very dry skin. Suppurating grooves in the nails. Psoriasis. Rheumatism.

A need for excitement in life.

Restlessness, nervousness at night.

Numbness, tingling in the upper limbs during sleep (pins and needles). Limbs go to sleep with tingling when sitting.

There are many rheumatic and gouty symptoms and scapular pains, both in the bones and joints.

Anxiety, and oppressed feeling in the chest.

Aversions: dislikes open air, indolence, and great aversion to exertion, either mental or physical, aversion to work, aversion to mental work, and to being spoken to.

The compositae family...

Bellis perennis (the daisy)

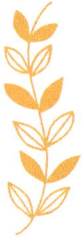

This is a plant remedy. It is made from the daisy. It is from the injury family (of the compositae family) of homeopathic remedies and has a sphere of action on cysts, and herpes. It can also be used as a 'blockbuster' anti-miasmatic remedy, to pave the way and open up the patient to the deeper disturbance which can then be treated constitutionally.

Akin to the trauma remedy *Arnica Montana* that is used to soothe muscle aches from sprains, strains and bruises, basically any system of the body where there has been leakage of blood, *Bellis Perennis* is used to balance extreme stressful sensitivity to injury, and with this an ability to trust again. This will in turn help local symptoms such as cysts and other skin conditions including acne, especially when they are related to an internal stress. *Bellis Perennis* is used in cases of trauma to the uterus, including the trauma of labour and caesarean section.

Bellis Perennis is a useful remedy for bruises, sprains, and injuries to the deeper tissues from surgery where Arnica has not acted.

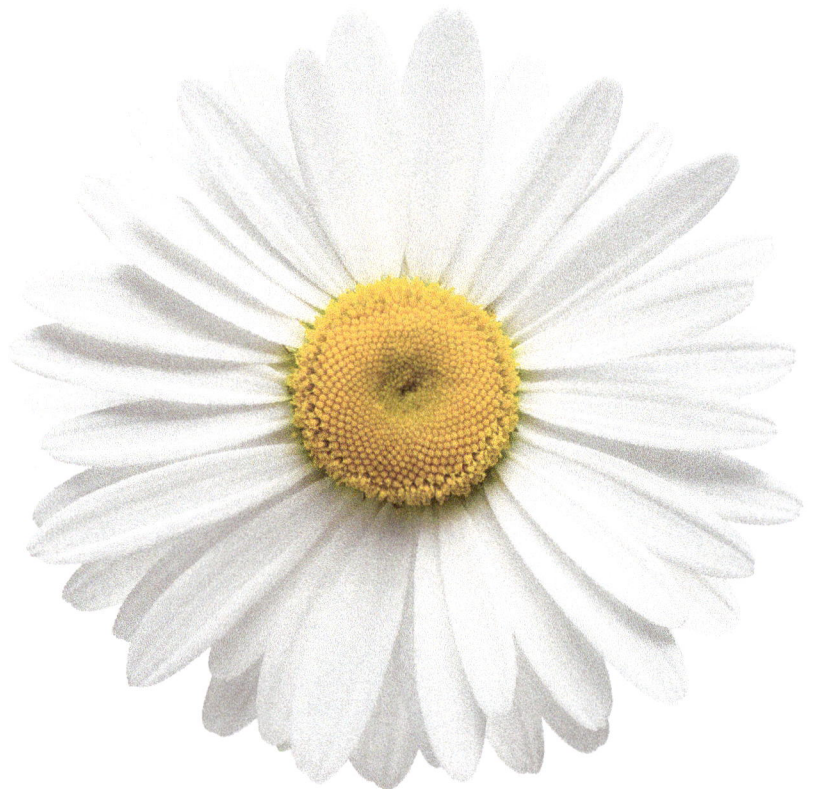

...Plant family remedies from the injury family.

Lappa arctium (Burdock)

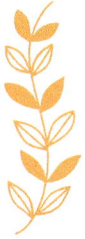

Lappa Arctium is a plant remedy made from Burdock. It is also from the injury family (of the compositae family) of homeopathic remedies and has its sphere of action on cysts, and is very important in skin therapeutics, in particular acne and eczema.

Lappa Arctium is a leading remedy for its action on the prolapse of uterus, characterised as an immensely sore bruised feeling in the uterus and apparently entire lack of tonicity of the pelvic contents. Symptoms are aggravated by standing, walking, or sudden jarring. Traditionally also useful for gonorrhoea, gout, impotence, leucorrhoea, rheumatism, ringworm, and ulcers.

THE MATRIDONALS (GIFTS OF THE MOTHER)

Pregnancy, birth, and development

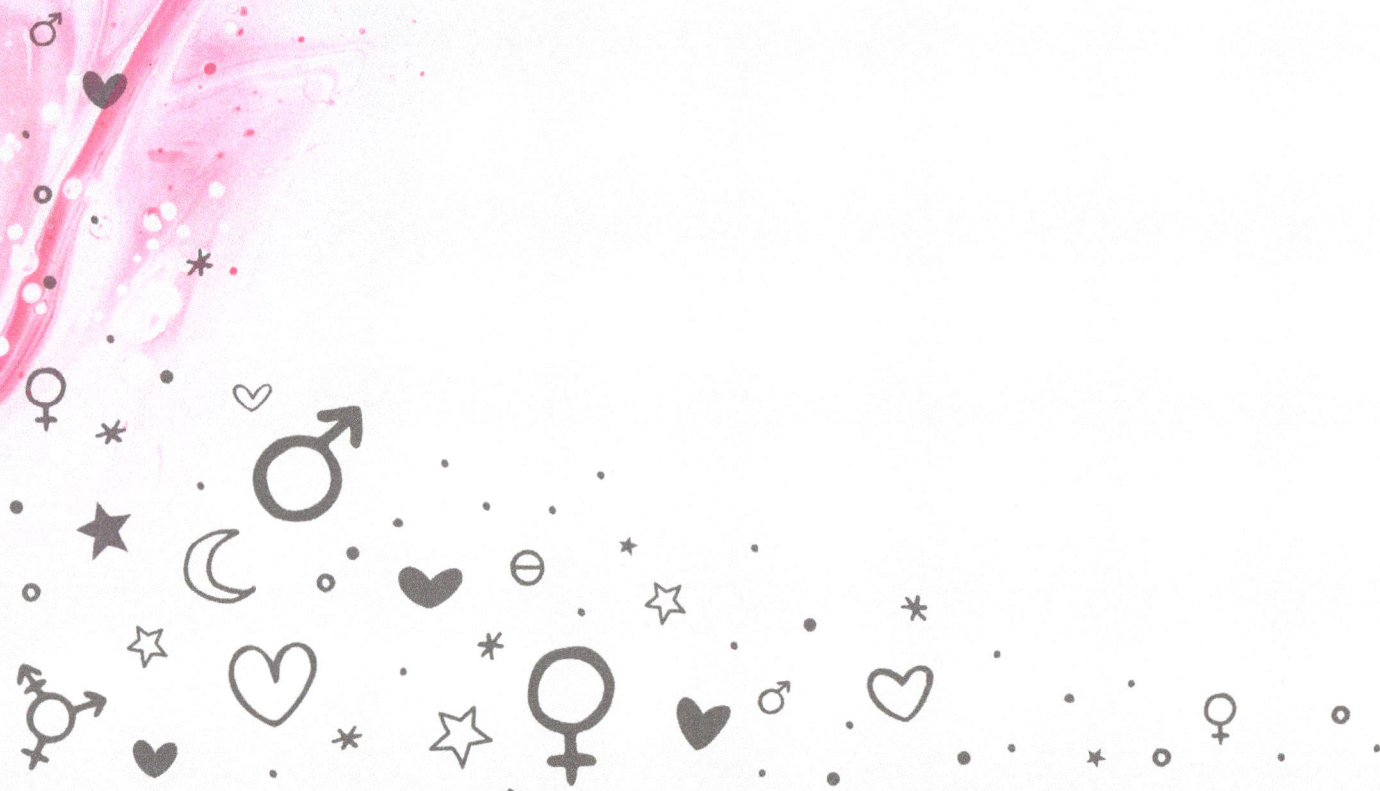

Chorda umbilicalis (Umbilical cord)

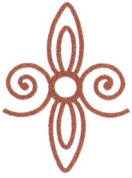

The main themes of umbilical cord are connection, letting go, release and breaking the bonds, growth and dimensions, and transformation.

There are problems with bonding; they cannot sever loveless ties; or have lost a vital bond.

The release of people and of life itself, feeling free to die. There is also a desire to be free from others, detach oneself from the group, to refuse to be influenced, and to stand up for oneself.

The connection is with mother earth, family, life, convictions and other situations, different from the connection with self.

Physical complaints include allergies, sneezing and reacting to everything.

Symptoms described in the *Materia Medica* relate to trituration performed with umbilical cord in the Hahnemann Institute in the Netherlands in 2007. During this process, the symptoms express themselves in stages, from the physical level to the mental, to the 4C, to the spiritual, to the 5C level. At this final stage, experiences transcend the earthly dimension.

Umbilical cord is a sarcode that closely relates to birth and early development. It belongs to this small group of remedies all related to pregnancy, birth and development.

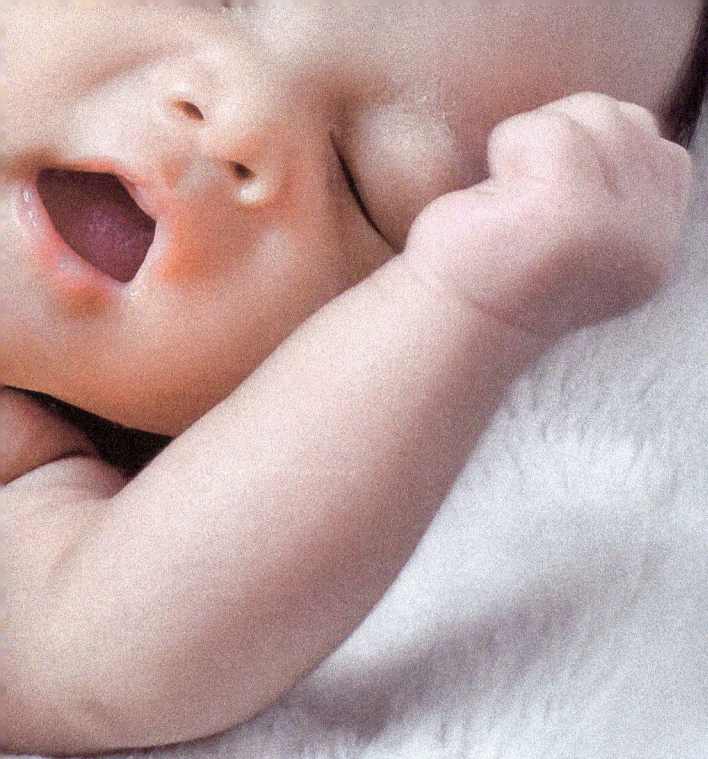

On Children

And a woman who held a babe against her bosom said, Speak to us of
    children. And he said;
Your children are not your children.
They are the sons and daughters of Life's longing for itself.
They come through you but not from you,
And though they are with you yet they belong not to you.
You may give them your love but not your thoughts,
For they have their own thoughts.
You may house their bodies but not their souls,
For their souls dwell in the house of tomorrow, which you cannot visit, not
    even in your dreams.
You may strive to be like them, but seek not to make them like you.
For life goes not backward nor tarries with yesterday.
You are the bows from which your children as living arrows are sent forth.
The archer sees the mark upon the path of the infinite, and He bends you with
    His might that His arrows may go swift and far.
Let your bending in the archer's hand be for gladness;
For even as He loves the arrow that flies, so He loves also the bow that is stable.

From 'The Prophet' by Kahlil Gibran.

Placenta humanum (Placenta)

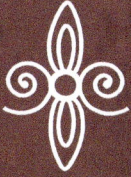

The physiology

The functions of the placenta play a huge role throughout pregnancy – it acts as the kidneys, lungs and intestines for the baby.

☾ Respiration and nutrition: The placenta enables the foetus to take oxygen and nutrients from the maternal blood.

☾ Excretion: It allows carbon dioxide and other waste products to pass from the foetus to the maternal circulatory system for excretion.

☾ Protection: It acts as a protective barrier between the foetus and infection, facilitating the transfer of antibodies. In addition, amniotic fluid provides a stable environment that protects the foetus from physical harm while still allowing free movement.

☾ Secretion: It excretes multiple hormones, including oestrogen and progesterone. The oestrogen prevents the pituitary gland from making follicle-stimulating hormone (FSH), which stimulates the ripening of the follicles in the ovary. The progesterone synchronises the growth of the uterus with the baby's development and prepares the breasts for milk production before the birth.

The anthropology

The placenta is the home for this spirit and soul for the next nine months. In Australia, the placenta is not an honoured organ and is usually disposed of efficiently; the final stage of labour, the delivery of the placenta, often has little importance and value. We must remember that the birth is not over until after this final stage, and the placenta has been delivered.

In different cultures, there is a huge importance placed on the whole birthing process and it begins right from the moment of conception; we can consider this when thinking about the journey of the soul. The soul connection is believed to be held in the placenta, as this is the channel through which the spirit journey continues. It is an extremely respected organ.

Some people perceive the placenta as the genetic 'sibling', as the placenta and the child have been living together in the womb for nine months. Many cultures support childbirth traditions where they honour the placenta and its role in pregnancy and childbirth. For some mothers, the way the placenta is treated after its delivery is almost as important as the way the child is treated.

The cutting of the cord takes place once the placenta has been delivered. When we understand the crucial role the placenta has played, it is easy to see what a symbolic act this is, and yet it is often done without much consideration.

Note: Scientific research has looked at the importance of placental/umbilical blood as a contribution to bone marrow transplants in the treatment of leukaemia. As research continues, the placenta is starting to play a more prominent role in our culture. Truth will always find a way.

The homeopathic remedy

The proving of this remedy was done at the Welsh College of Homeopathy, United Kingdom.

The symptoms that *placenta humanum* would be prescribed for also include, but are not limited to:

☾ A desire for and awareness of beauty. Having a desire to touch and wear pearls.

☾ Conscientious of everything being in order; having an aversion to untidiness.

☾ They have an inability to dance and to get into the rhythm.

☾ Healthy. Nails are strong and grow quickly. Skin and hair glow, similar to during pregnancy.

☾ Spots and blotches. Blotchy rash on chest and upper arms and spreading to back; this is slightly irritating. There are spots on the forehead, potentially acne suppressed by antibiotics in teens.

☾ Wounds are slow to heal.

☾ Personal journey and strengthening of the individual. Realisation, awareness, recognition, re-awakening, purpose, strengthening, individual, potential, acceptance, clearing out, resolving old issues, healing of chronic symptoms, letting go, cutting ties.

☾ Feeling like they can't handle impulses, resulting in anxiety and restlessness.

The colour

The colour theme running through this remedy is burgundy. Red also comes up. It's interesting to note that the overall colour of the placenta is dull red (with a thin grey). Red is also the colour of the base/root chakra, the seat of self-awareness and foundation for life. The root chakra helps us to strengthen our essential connection to mother earth and feel grounded and 'rooted' in life. It is responsible for the basic needs of security and stability, confidence and strength, with the related emotions being fear or courage.

In addition, it has been noted that burgundy is the colour formed by mixing the colours red and violet, the colours of the root and crown chakras.

Keynotes

Disconnection from roots

Lack of connection from roots and source are dominant symptoms

Lac humanum/maternum
(Human mother's milk)
Difficult digestion of life and food

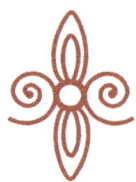

There is a slight difference between the two remedies
Lac humanum and *Lac maternum*. *Maternum* is made from
colostrum and the *humanum* is made from regular mother's
milk. Both have different provings and albeit similar have a
few differences.

Breastmilk contains a lot of proteins, including antibodies,
and is the ideal temperature for human consumption.
Colostrum precedes the production of milk. It is the yellowish
fluid secreted in the first few hours or days after giving birth
and consists mainly of lymphocytes and immunoglobulins.
Breastfeeding promotes the physical and emotional contact
between mother and child. Because of this, mother's milk is
preferable to artificial feeding. Milk is considered the best
biological fluid for optimal infant growth and development.

Region: Mucous membranes (mouth, throat, stomach) and
female reproductive organs. (This relates to *Lac humanum* –
the regions that the medicine works on healing.)

The essence of Lac maternum
The main theme running through *maternum* is incarnation
into current life. Incarnation that takes place during pregnancy
is seemingly not concluded at birth and the mother's milk
helps to gently bring the baby down.

Some of the physical complaints: Skin diseases especially
eczema and psoriasis, energy too high in the physical body
(associated with the lack of incarnation) and creates headache,
migraine, dizziness, vertigo, empty feeling, loss of hair.

There is a deep unawareness of their true identity that comes
from this lack of incarnation. The *Lac maternum* patient is not
centred, they are easily disconnected and influenced by the
energy of the surrounding people. They do not have clarity
of mind, and are often confused.

Keynotes

Lacks humanity

Sadness during the
letdown of milk

Hormone imbalances

Want for confidence

Lack of nurturing by
the mother

Not in body

Physically awkward,
Clumsy

Non-spatial

Ungrounded

Feels alone; forsaken;
isolated; neglected,
lacks concentration;
detached, alienated, yet
with heightened senses

Leading guiding symptoms to prescribe Lac humanum

O A need for control and to put the world close to home in order; untidiness is aggravating.

O Indifference to everything, feeling detached and feeling indifference to the suffering of others.

O A sense of isolation.

O Dreams about babies and death.

O Independence versus dependence. The dependent state is characterised by a desire to have something in the mouth (e.g. thumb-sucking); there is periodical desire to clamber onto mother's lap and to cuddle. They might also exhibit regressive behaviour.

O Eating disorders and huge fluctuations in body weight.

O Desire for sweet and/or warm things, such as chocolate or ginger.

O An aversion to sour foods.

O Desire for salt.

O Increased appetite.

O Menstrual blood is dark brown or nearly black.

Lac humanum brings empathy and puts us directly into our bodies, helping our soul to incorporate itself into our physical being. All of the matridonal remedies have this facet, but it is most apparent with breastmilk.

Amniota humana (Amniotic fluid)

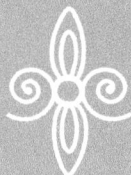

This remedy is traditionally used to help take the patient back to the place where they were formed, connecting them back to the womb, including any trauma that occurred during gestation. The amniotic fluid sheds light on how you were formed and what was going on during your formation.

It is indicated when the physical health history of the patient includes birth trauma, preterm delivery, lack of mothering, and lack of breastfeeding.

The functions of the matridonal tissues (sarcode remedies) are to help give the spirit a sense of bodily self, and physical boundaries that contribute to representing oneself. They are also indicated when there is:

· Spaciness, ungroundedness, poor balance, or a floaty feeling.

· Feelings of isolation or a lack of connection to humanity.

· Lacking empathy, not feeling 'human', feeling very different from others.

· Feeling as if "Life has never started for me" or "I wish I could start over".

Useful for children and adults alike, the use of matridonal remedies in classical homeopathy must always fit the symptoms of the entire case. This includes key mental and emotional factors, as well as the indicators surrounding birth, conception and breastfeeding, and any physical or emotional traumas associated with that point in time.

In my opinion, these homeopathic remedies are safe for children, pregnant women, right through to the elderly. I remind people that with homeopathy, we are not adding anything here – we are working with the body's own tendency towards healing. It is an energetic medicine. We are not changing the chemical composition of the body; the remedies stimulate the body's own energy flow and gives it a gentle nudge to heal itself. In effect, the remedy does not cure, the body does so itself.

As for the alcohol, when prescribing for pregnant women and children, or even highly sensitive types, we use the pillules. There is no alcohol in the pillules.

You can transform
your wounding
into your medicine.

Mastitis

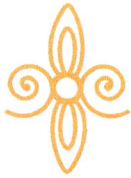

Symptoms of mastitis include sore breasts and inflammation, which can lead to an abscess. It is usually unilateral. Symptoms include painful lumps, tenderness, redness, heat and flu-like feelings. It can be caused by improper positioning or long delays between feeds. Blocked ducts can be caused by dry secretions over nipple openings. It should be treated ASAP with bedrest, fluids and cabbage leaves. Continue nursing, and you can seek out breastfeeding counselling.

Homeopathic remedies for mastitis, and their guiding symptoms, include:

Belladonna: Rapid onset. Fiery hot feelings, intense fever and red-streaked breasts.

Bryonia: Slow onset pains. Aggravated from slightest of motion, aggravated by heat. Accompanied by great thirst.

Phytolacca: Radiating pain over the whole body. Mastitis after mental or emotional stress. Hard and sensitive with purple hue. Painful, lumpy breasts.

Lac-c: Alternating sides. Dries up milk. Painful nipples.

Silica: Stitching pains, splinter-like abscesses. Blocked ducts. Pulsatilla if very teary.

Castor equi: Cracked, sore nipples, excessively tender. Swelling of breasts. Violent itching in breasts; are reddened.

Other considerations: Graphites, hepar sulph, sulphur, mercury.

Borax (bicarb soda): Pain in opposite breast when child nurses. Empty feeling in breasts after child nurses, with stitches, compressing with pressure of hand ameliorates. Milk is cheesy and bad. Child refuses milk.

Other considerations: Bryonia, castor equi, graphites.

Newborns

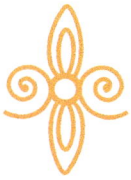

Newborns can have thrush if the mother has had antibiotics during labour.

Remedy: Borax (bicarb soda)

Indications: White-coated tongue. Startles when put down in cot. This remedy is used for great anxiety from downward motion; when laying the child down on a couch or in the crib, cries and clings to the nurse; when rocking, dancing, swinging; going down stairs, or rapidly downhill.

Remedies for newborns are best facilitated by breastfeeding post-delivery; it is a really nice, gentle, and diluted way for your newborn baby to be treated. That which created it, will always do well from the same remedy! In fact, the entire family living in the same environment will benefit from the same remedy the baby is prescribed! Other methods of administering remedies to newborns are in a bath or via the skin when safe and appropriate to do so.

DIRECTIONS OF CURE

A tool in homeopathic therapeutics

'Hering's Law' by Dr Constantine Hering; Germany 1800

As described to the 1845 American edition of The Chronic Diseases by Samuel Hahnemann. (9, Appendix 2)

Under the action of the similar remedy, healing takes place and symptoms move in three directions:

From above, downwards: For example, head symptoms will go first, and action moves downwards, causing symptoms to arise further down the body, particularly down the limbs.

From within, outwards: For example, to the skin, urine, faeces, mucus linings. From the more inwards organs to the more outward, eg from liver to bowel, from lungs to skin.

In the reverse order of arrival: For example, the most recent symptoms disappear first, and less recent symptoms will reappear and be treated with the same or another remedy. It often happens that the first remedy will ease the current presenting symptoms, and old symptoms will reappear. Then they will also disappear and others will come up, one at a time, dating back to childhood, going away without any need for intervention from other treatments. This is true deep healing taking place.

CONSULTATIONS

Here are a few more ideas I often share with my patients...

♈ When we dismiss our body's signs and symptoms, it drives the discord inward, to a deeper organ, making it more difficult to treat and potentially more dangerous. The body will always find another valve to express itself when we don't look at the symptoms it is presenting us with.

♈ Instead of using medicated topicals for a skin condition, I would prescribe a constitutional remedy to stop it coming up in the first place. We are prescribing at the baseline here.

♈ Do I need to take a supplement? Prescribing constitutionally is beneficial because once the baseline is stable, I would expect vitamin and mineral levels to be better as well.

♈ The baseline shift will percolate to the physicals.

♈ How do cortisone drugs suppress susceptibility? Cortisone will suppress your susceptibility to respond to homeopathic remedies. No matter how well indicated they will not do their job. Homeopathic cortisone can be given in this case to re-engage the susceptibility of the body to respond.

♈ Other suppressants used for skin conditions include Tacrolimus. This is an immuno-suppressant and opposes the effects of the homeopathic process.

It's important all medicating creams are stopped otherwise the homeopathic cortisone can't start the healing process while the two processes are confusing the body while opposing each other. The patient must decide what they really want.

DISCOVER MORE

Silica/Silicea (pure flint)

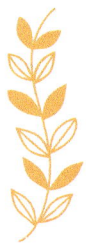

Derived from quartz or flint

Silica is a great remedy for skin issues, as it is necessary for collagen formation and collagen is necessary for healthy skin.

Silica can be used as a homeopathic preparation or taken from tissue salts. Tissue salts are an alternative chewable tablet that can be taken daily. Remember, most skin conditions (apart from contact dermatitis) arise from internal problems which must be treated. Therefore, tissue salts are suitable as an acute remedy for localised temporary natural relief. They are working at what we call 'stage one' (the localised symptoms) and can absolutely be taken alongside your homeopath-prescribed remedy, as they will not interfere with a constitutional remedy (although it is not recommended for pregnant women or people with pacemakers). This means that you can get relief while we work on the deeper stuff at the baseline!

MATERIA MEDICA

The homeopathic preparation silica in potency 6x or 30 – used for acute skin conditions where injuries won't heal. Cracks, bed sores, abscesses, profuse offensive sweat.

Silica is considered the homeopathic scalpel and is not recommended for pregnant women or people with pacemakers. Silica helps the body expel splinters, kidney stones, papules, stools and infection from the wound site.

Constitutionally prescribed for people with a chilly disposition; symptoms are worse in the cold.

The silica patient is yielding, faint-hearted, anxious, and sensitive to all impressions.

There is difficulty in absorption and digestion of food or nutrients by the body and consequent defective nutrition.

Arnica montana (Wolf's bane)

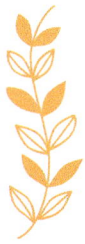

From the plant kingdom

In acute prescribing, this remedy is the first to consider for aching or strained muscles that are worsened by touch, motion, cold and damp weather conditions, or after overexertion. It can also be used for a black eye and inflammation from external injuries.

Arnica is produced from Wolf's bane. It is especially suited to cases when an injury has caused the presenting complaint. Often prescribed after traumatic injuries, overuse of any organ or strains, it is used as a muscular tonic when the limbs and body ache as if beaten and joints feel as if they're sprained.

MATERIA MEDICA

Patients requiring Arnica fear the approach of anyone. There has been traumatism of grief, remorse, or sudden realisation of financial loss; they may have experienced a mental strain or shock. The whole body is very sensitive and they feel a desire to be left alone.

It is of dictatorial nature, speaking with an air of command. There is a great sensitivity and aversion to intrusion; "Don't touch me!" It has been a very beneficial remedy for those who take the stance of a military officer because of the psyche and structure of this medicine and individuals of this nature.

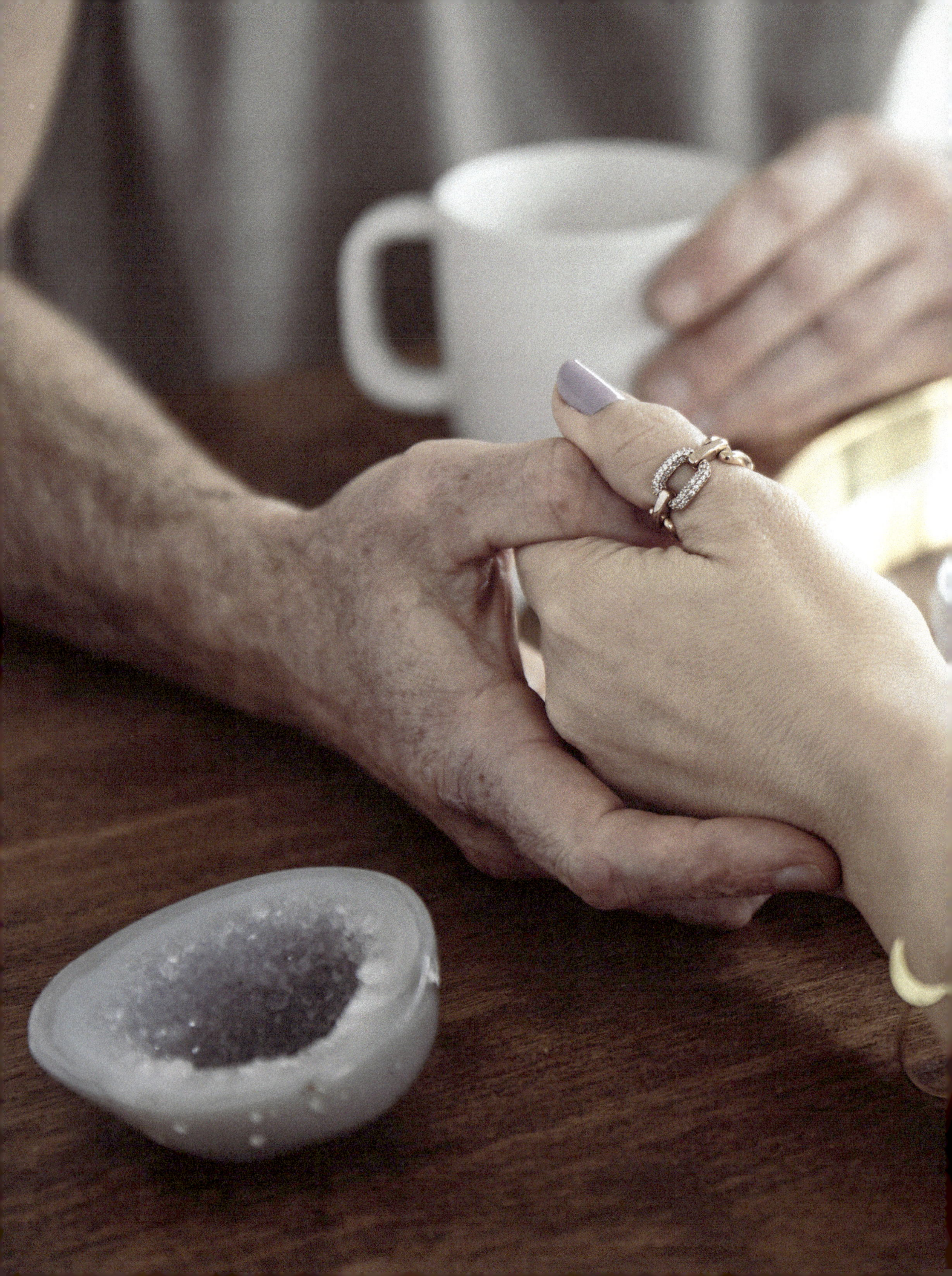

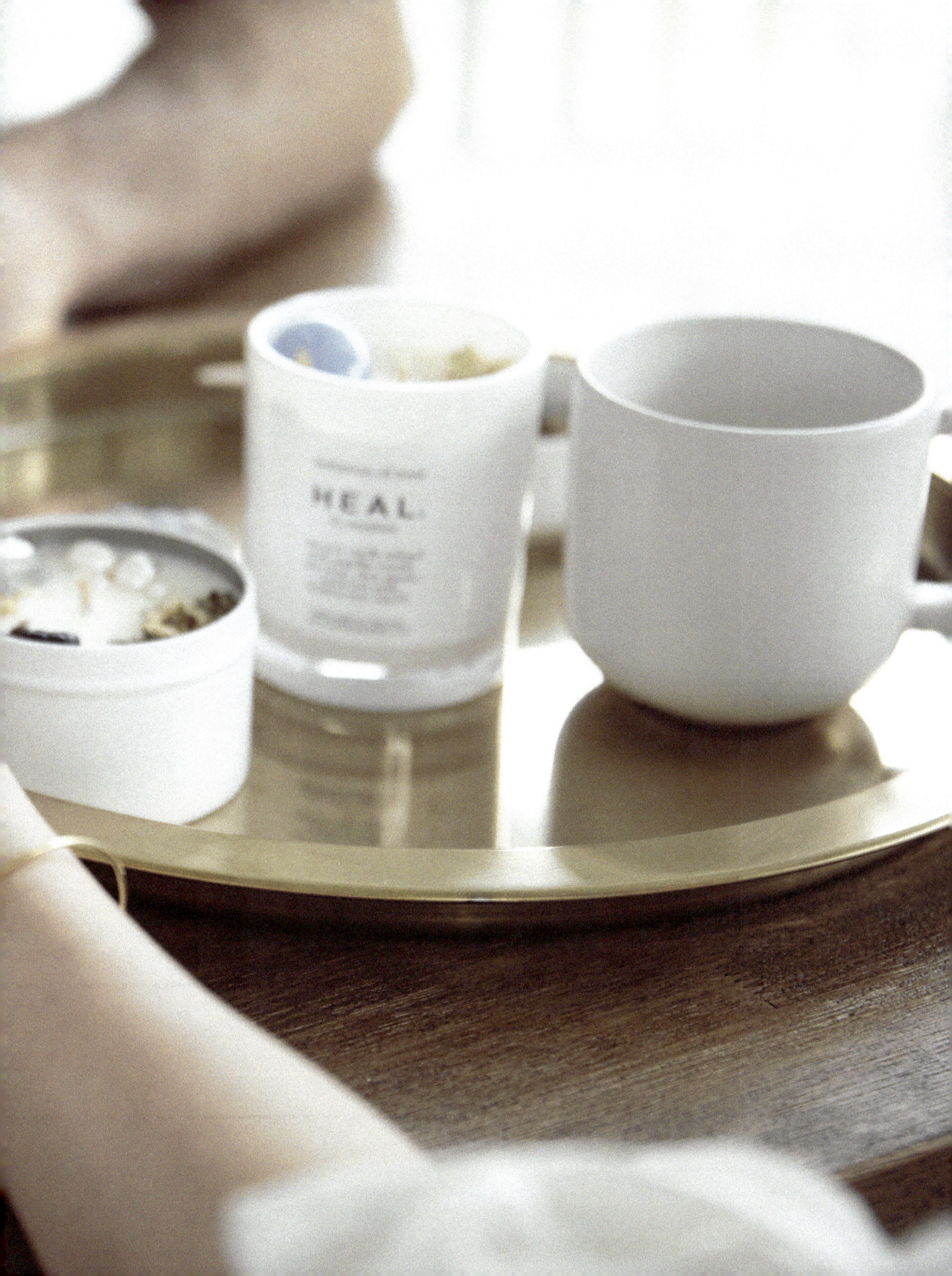

HEAL.

THE MIASMS

"Every constitution is predisposed by his miasm to express a certain pattern of symptomatology in every disease he suffers."

– Samuel Hahnemann

When studying chronic disease, it was concluded that the most important awareness was that most symptoms almost always begin at the level of the skin and mucous membrane. Symptoms then proceeded inwards when the skin symptoms were suppressed. Hahnemann later referred to this as the "dyscrasia of modern medicine".

Hahnemann theorised that these initial suppressions were the fundamental cause of most chronic diseases which followed. The causation of a range of different diseases and ailments which man suffered from was called the miasm.

His experiments identified three groups of skin manifestations:

Psora: A group of diseases which followed an initial 'itch' symptom on skin.

Sycosis: A group of diseases which followed treatment of a symptom on skin that was a gonorrhoeal discharge or wart.

Syphilis: A group of diseases which followed initial treatment on skin that was a syphilitic chancre.

Every disease could have either one or a combination of more miasmatic patterns or could have a progression of specific patterns, e.g. psora to sycosis to syphilis.

MATERIA MEDICA

Tubercular: Traced to skin conditions/
chronic inflammations which are
characterised by suppuration, pus formation,
abscesses with tendency to bleed easily.

Cancer: Fastidiousness, exaggerated
precision.

Strong sense of rhythm, love of dancing and
sensitivity to music which can make them cry.

Fears: of cancer, disease, death. Prolonged
fear, unhappiness and despairs recovery.

Anticipation: Anguish, e.g. late arrival of
husband, child, failing exams.

Sympathetic to others.

Sensitivity to reprimand.

Leprosy: Intense oppression, intense
hopelessness, isolation and an intense desire
for change. Disgust.

Carcinosinum

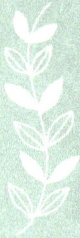

Carcinosinum is made from breast cancer tissue. This remedy is a nosode and shows a picture of the cancer miasm, said to be an equal proportion of three other miasms mixed.

Appearance

☆ The carcinosinum patient will appear with pale or (milk) coffee-coloured skin.

☆ The sclera is blue.

☆ There is grimacing or constant blinking of the eyes.

☆ Lots of moles, naevi. Especially black macules.

☆ Inverted nipples.

Family history

There is a high incidence of cancer, tuberculosis, diabetes, leukaemia, or pernicious anaemia through the family.

Tip: when there is a family history of cancer, carcinosinum can often heal insomnia.

Personal history

★ Often these patients are "never well since...".

★ Severe incidence of whooping cough (these patients do very well on carcinosinum), croup, glandular fever, pneumonia, rheumatic fever, bronchitis, pox diseases, anorexia nervosa, herpes I and II, vaccinations.

★ Lots of coughs, colds, flu, sore throat and inflammatory disease.

★ Recurrent swollen glands.

★ History of migraines.

★ Chronic acid stomach conditions.

★ The dual experience of any childhood disease or after adolescence.

Keynotes

The lead remedy for chronic fatigue syndrome.

Perfectionism

It's about what other people will think. They have to be seen to be perfect.

The situation of carcinosinum is that of a child with a strict upbringing. The parents insist that the child should be perfect. These children have good manners, they behave themselves and are not mischievous. The carcinosinum patient is heavily controlled by the person on who they depend.

They are very conscious of good taste and desire perfection in everything. Being neat and clean is not enough; it must be perfect and they are neurotic about it.

◇ Related to the desire for perfection and a sensitive nature makes them very sensitive to reprimands.

◇ Also out of this comes anticipatory anxiety. If they organise a party, they are not so much concerned that the party should get going as that everything should be perfect. Sometimes this can be so extreme that they become suicidal.

◇ There is a high degree of seriousness and commitment; there is an easy assumption of guilt.

◇ Extremes of fastidiousness, earnestness, responsibility and over-conscientiousness or untidiness.

Sensitive emotionally

☽ Sensitive to reproach, easily offended.

☽ Dislikes consolation. There is sadness but they cannot cry.

☽ Aversion or aggravation from conversation.

☽ Sympathy and anxiety about others. They are caring and concerned for others; they are friendly, sociable and cheerful people who always come to me smiling. They will tell their doctor that they feel better even though they are worse, as they feel sympathy for the doctor and do not want to offend.

Repression of feelings

❈ They accept everything with a kind of resignation and it all accumulates inside without any expression to the outside world. They have a lot of grief but are very yielding.

❈ There is suppressed resentment or anger.

❈ Prolonged emotional states – fear or sadness, resentment or anger.

❈ Someone in the family "makes me sick".

Desires stimulation

❏ Enjoy watching thunderstorms.

❏ Very sensitive to music, flowing motion and they love dancing. Dancing becomes their survival mechanism.

❏ Artistic disposition – music, dance, painting, literature and poetry. Nature lovers.

The secret

The carc patient's secrets may be incest, child abuse, the baby of their mother's affair.

Anxiety and fears

○ Great anxiety; anticipation. "Today is the tomorrow I agonised over yesterday, here it is and I'm fine."

○ Fear of disease, especially cancer.

○ Full of fears (cancer, contamination) which are prolonged and sit in the stomach. They pull the skin around the edge of their nails or bite their nails.

Desires and aversions

Strong in the carc patient is the desire or aversion to chocolate, egg, salt, fat, fruit, meat, butter, or sweets.

Generally

✱ There is weakness and fatigue.

✱ Alternation of symptoms; one side of the body to the other.

✱ Ill effects of vaccination.

✱ Strongly influenced by the sea air.

✱ Children with recurrent fevers and inflammation.

✱ Wounds are slow to heal.

✱ Symptoms are changeable.

Sleep

The child lies in bed on knees with their head on the pillow. This is very characteristic of carcinosinum, yet all the nosodes have this common trait.

LAW OF ATTRACTION VERSUS SURRENDER

HEAL. is the secret ingredient to manifesting our desires.

Fifteen years ago, when I first bought the book *The Secret* by Rhonda Byrne and started visualising, believing and saying affirmations, I wish someone had told me the real secret.

After all of that work, I was convinced my dreams were 'coming' ... only they never came! That is, until I started to understand the key component that would unlock everything: HEAL.

Listening to (well-meaning) self-help 'gurus' tell me that I just needed to stay positive to achieve my dreams became nauseatingly annoying. I was trying to do this work, and it was when I was training to be a homeopath that the lightbulb moment came, and I really started to understand that the pain never expressed is what causes disease.

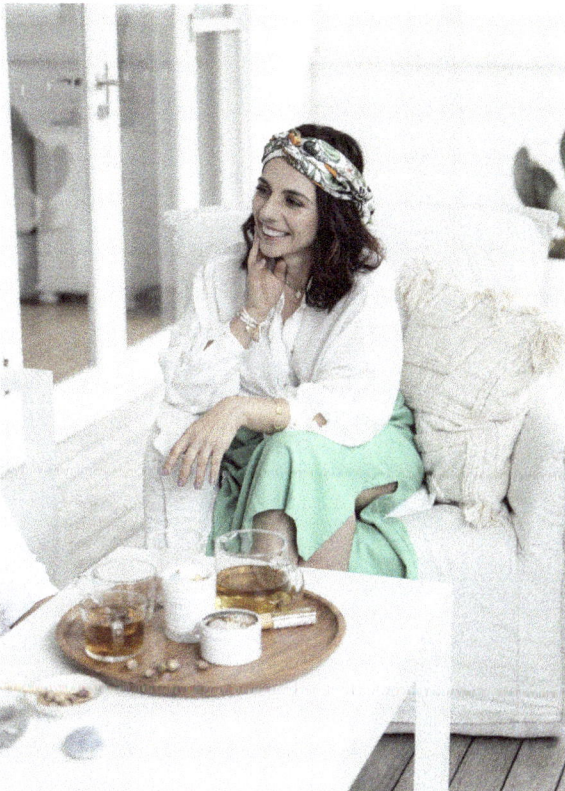

Avoidance of pain and distress is an unhealthy compensatory mechanism and is a form of limitation and disease. Acknowledging and appreciating the pain and distress is a way to release it and it's an important part of healing.

Suppression of symptoms or emotions will drive the discord deeper within. True healing is being able to experience both extremes of one's polarity – pain and pleasure – and being able to bounce back to equilibrium without being stuck in either. The homeopathic process is one way of achieving this.

A feeling of equanimity develops as the central nervous system is free from the trauma response, it is finally safe to get what we want, and the physical symptoms disappear.

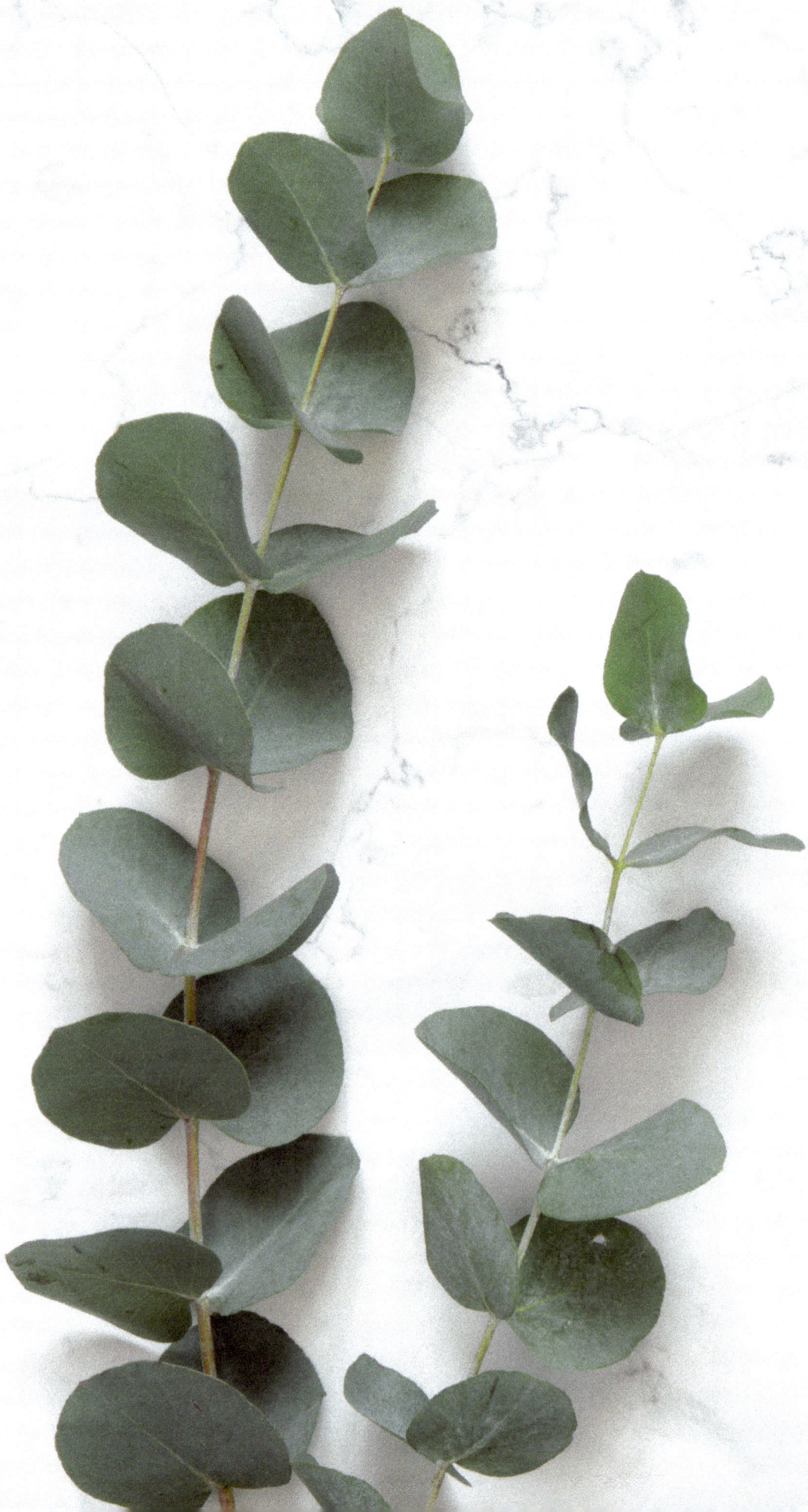

You won't heal
pretending
you're not hurt.

Thuja occidentalis
(Northern white-cedar or Arborvitae)

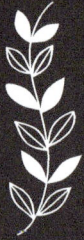

Traditionally, the main action of Thuja has been on the skin and genito-urinary organs. Thuja affects the blood, skin, gastrointestinal and respiratory tracts, and organs such as the kidneys and brain.

All effects are worse for damp and better for warmth. It is used for the hydrogenoid constitution who is chilly with predominantly left-sided complaints. They commonly have dark bags under their eyes, a pale waxy and dirty looking face, foul and acrid foot sweats and yellow staining sweat.

Mentally they are very anxious and disoriented. This is mainly an antipsychotic remedy. In homeopathy, 'psychotic' does not have the same meaning as in conventional medicine. In homeopathy, one of the miasms is called 'psychotic', and it has nothing to do with the psychosis seen in conventional diagnosis.

Keynotes

Ill-humoured. Great prostration; sad; loathes life.

Mind and body feel separate.

Sensation as if something live is in the abdomen.

Tearing head pain, or pain like a nail in the head.

Wart-like excrescences upon mucous and cutaneous surfaces. Fig warts and genital warts.

Fixed ideas.

Vacancy in head, with inability to think.

Numbness in brain.

Slow speech with frequent interruption, because of feeling obliged to hunt for words.

Emotional sensitiveness; music causes weeping and trembling.

Vertigo when closing the eyes, then it is immediately better on opening the eyes again.

Insane women will not be touched or approached.

White scaly dandruff; hair is dry and falling out.

Restlessness.

Great depression.

They will meditate over every tiff, with anxious concern for the future.

Sensation as if the body is brittle and could break as if made of glass.

Sleep disturbances; wakes at 3 am; dreams of devils and of failing.

Fishy odour of discharges.

Sunspots in the aged.

It is better for warmth, free secretions, motion, crossing legs, touch, wrapping up, and fresh air.

It is worse for the cold, damp weather, when urinating, and during sunrise to sunset (3 am to 3 pm).

Homeopathic cortisone

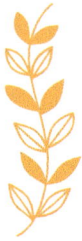

Homeopathic cortisone is prepared from cortisone. It is diluted and succussed in line with all homeopathic preparations. This is a way of chelating (detoxing) the residual toxic effects of the drug. In homeopathy, this is called isopathy, giving the same substance as what caused the malady. It is used often for first aid cases or to detoxify heavy metals or other toxic substances.

I give homeopathic cortisone in a triple split dose, then wait and watch for the response. I like to give it the time it needs to do its work, waiting, watching and redosing only when the action stops.

In my experience, a detox remedy can take any time from a few weeks to a few months to complete its job, depending on the level of suppression. They are deeply healing miasmatic remedies rather than superficial remedies, because they remove a complete disease complex layer (an extra level of disease caused by a medication that suppresses symptoms) that has been formed by the suppressive drug, triggering a baseline miasm.

Suppressants include steroid cortisone taken orally, as well as cortisone creams. Tacrolimus is another suppressant used. It's not a steroid, but it is an immunosuppressant and opposes the effects of the homeopathic process. I would prescribe homeopathic cortisone in this case to re-engage the susceptibility of the body to respond.

It is important all creams are stopped, otherwise the homeopathic cortisone can't start the healing process, as the two processes are confusing the body because they oppose each other.

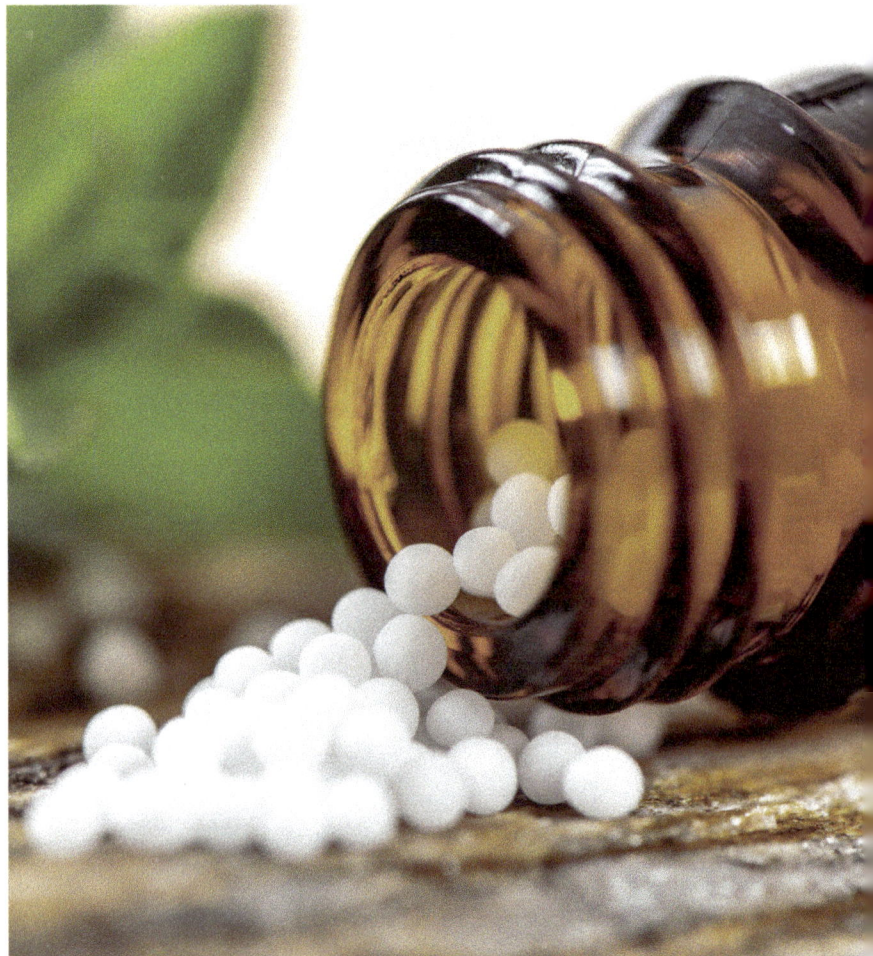

Sulphur (Sublimated sulphur)

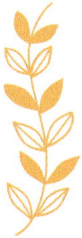

This is the great Hahnemannian antipsoric. Its action is from within outward, having an elective affinity for the skin. For more than 2000 years, sulphur has been found to be a most efficacious remedy against the itch.

MATERIA MEDICA

The sulphur patient produces heat and burning, with itching, made worse by heat of the bed.

Keynotes:

- Very forgetful.
- Constant heat on top of head.
- Adapted to those experiencing scrofulous diathesis (swollen glands due to disease).
- Those who are anxious, short-tempered, and quick to act.
- Plethoric, overflowing with excess energy.
- Skin particularly sensitive to changes in the air.
- Poor healing; infects easily.
- For those who sit, stand, or walk with hunched shoulders.
- Sulphur patients find standing uncomfortable; they struggle to stand at all, as every upright position causes discomfort.
- Unclean individuals, susceptible to skin infections.
- A complete loss of or excessive appetite, worse at 11 am.
- Food tastes too salty.
- Milk disagrees, as does meat.
- Great desire for sweets, alcohol and fats.
- Aversion to washing or being washed; always feel worse after bathing.
- Too lazy to rouse himself; too unhappy to live.
- Children cannot tolerate being washed or bathed.
- Emaciated, big-bellied, restless, hot, kicks off clothes at night, has worms.
- Complaints that are continually relapsing; patients seem to get almost well again then the disease returns, time and time again.

Traditionally, when other relevant remedies fail to produce a favourable effect, especially when illness is severe, sulphur serves to awaken the system, clearing up the case.

They are worse for suppressions, bathing, milk, heat of bed, heat, speaking, 11 am and the full moon.

Better for open air, warm applications, sweating, dry heat.

Matricaria chamomilla (German chamomile)

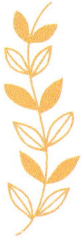

Chamomile can help irritability and pain intolerance. Chamomile is most often used in the second stage of irritability and pain intolerance – in other words, not in the infancy stages of the issue. Indications are of great irritability that is uncharacteristic to the patient and is caused by the intensity of the pain.

MATERIA MEDICA

Typically, the chamomilla patient becomes very irritable and fractious, orders people out of the room and might even have a temper tantrum. It has traditionally been used for any condition where this irritability is present.

Chamomilla is sensitive, irritable, thirsty, hot and numb. Oversensitiveness from abuse of coffee and narcotics. Pains are unendurable, associated with numbness. There are also night sweats.

In my experience, chamomilla is a brilliant remedy for babies when they're teething. It's often the first remedy to consider for unbearable pain, when the child is fretful, angry and inconsolable. The child might have one red cheek while the other is pale. The child can only be quietened when carried about and petted constantly.

Keynotes:

- Irritable from the pain.
- Whining restlessness. Child wants things which he refuses again.
- Diarrhoea during teething.
- Extreme sensitivity; wants to be carried; nervous; mind must be kept busy; averse to being spoken to; quarrelsome, angry, disagreeable, intolerant of pain.
- Rheumatic pains which drive them out of bed at night.
- Sensitive to all smells; coryza of the nose, with inability to sleep.
- Ringing in the ears. Earache with soreness; swelling and heat driving patient frantic.
- Dry, hacking cough which is worse from 9 pm to midnight and better for cold applications.
- Tongue is yellow with a bitter taste.
- Teething where the mentals fit; screams with unbearable pain between 9 pm and midnight.
- Unbearable colic; doubles up with the pain; flatulence which has a foul smell. Stools are hot, green, watery and slimy, like chopped spinach.

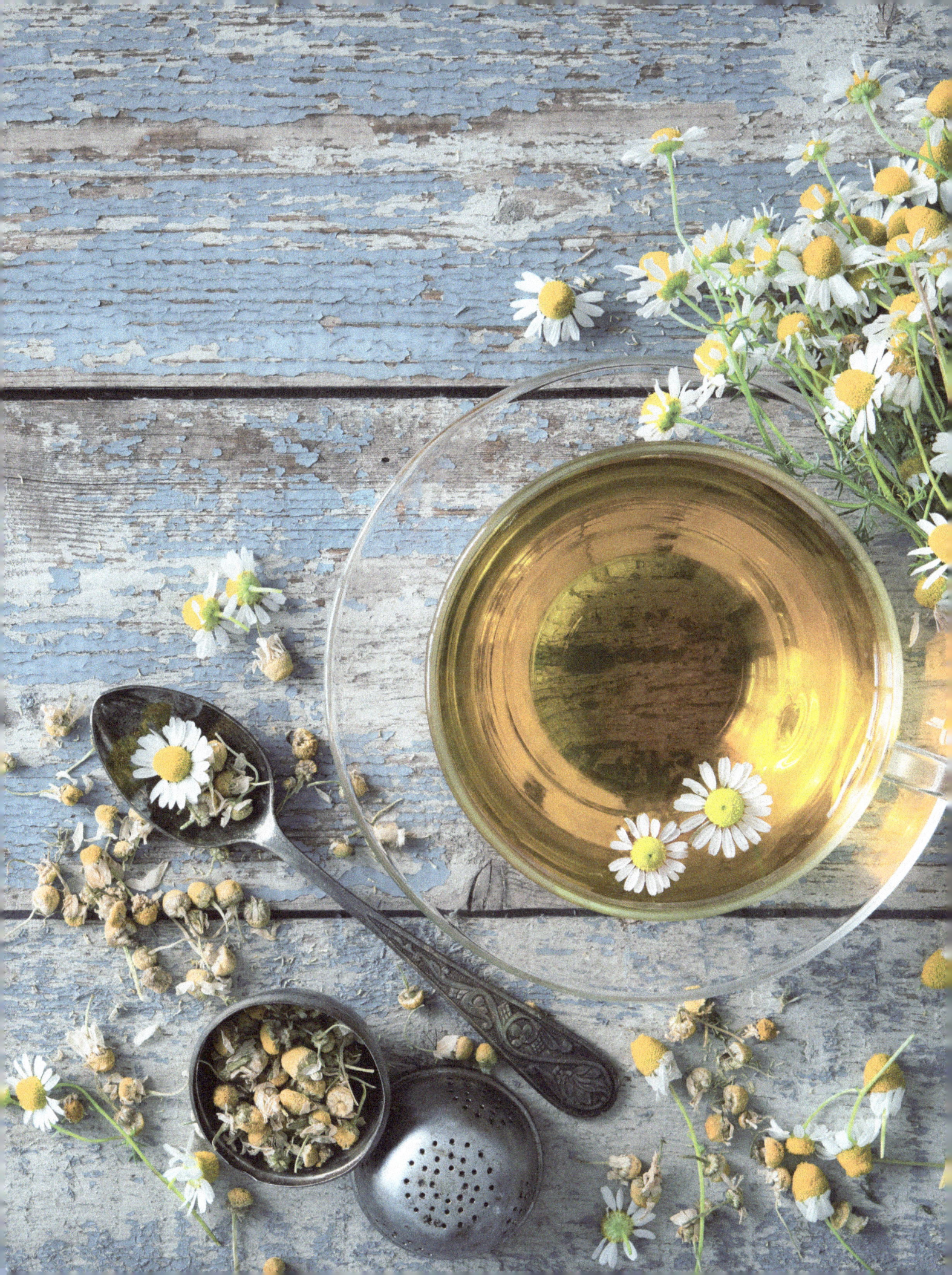

KINGDOMS IN HOMEOPATHY

Homeopathic remedies are sourced from nature and are largely categorised into three kingdoms: plants, animals and minerals. As we match different parts of your state and gain momentum through the different remedies, often patients find they have expressions of all three kingdoms at some point in their lives. I will prescribe on the peculiar symptoms of the presenting state.

Understanding the animal kingdom

The core essence of the issue in the animal patient is survival. This is seen through comparison and competition; only the strongest will be successful and live, the others will fail and die. Animals are inherent communicators; they use communication and social interaction as a way to survive and thrive in the wild. Attracting attention is the most innate need and important component of the animal's competitive persona. The animal patient will often display lively communication, sexuality, and attractiveness with a desire to be the centre of attention. Patients requiring an animal remedy will dress and behave in order to attract and be noticed. Hierarchy is another chief indicator of persons expressing themselves from the animal kingdom; they feel that others are superior or inferior to them, and see hierarchy and threats as a core element to their very existence.

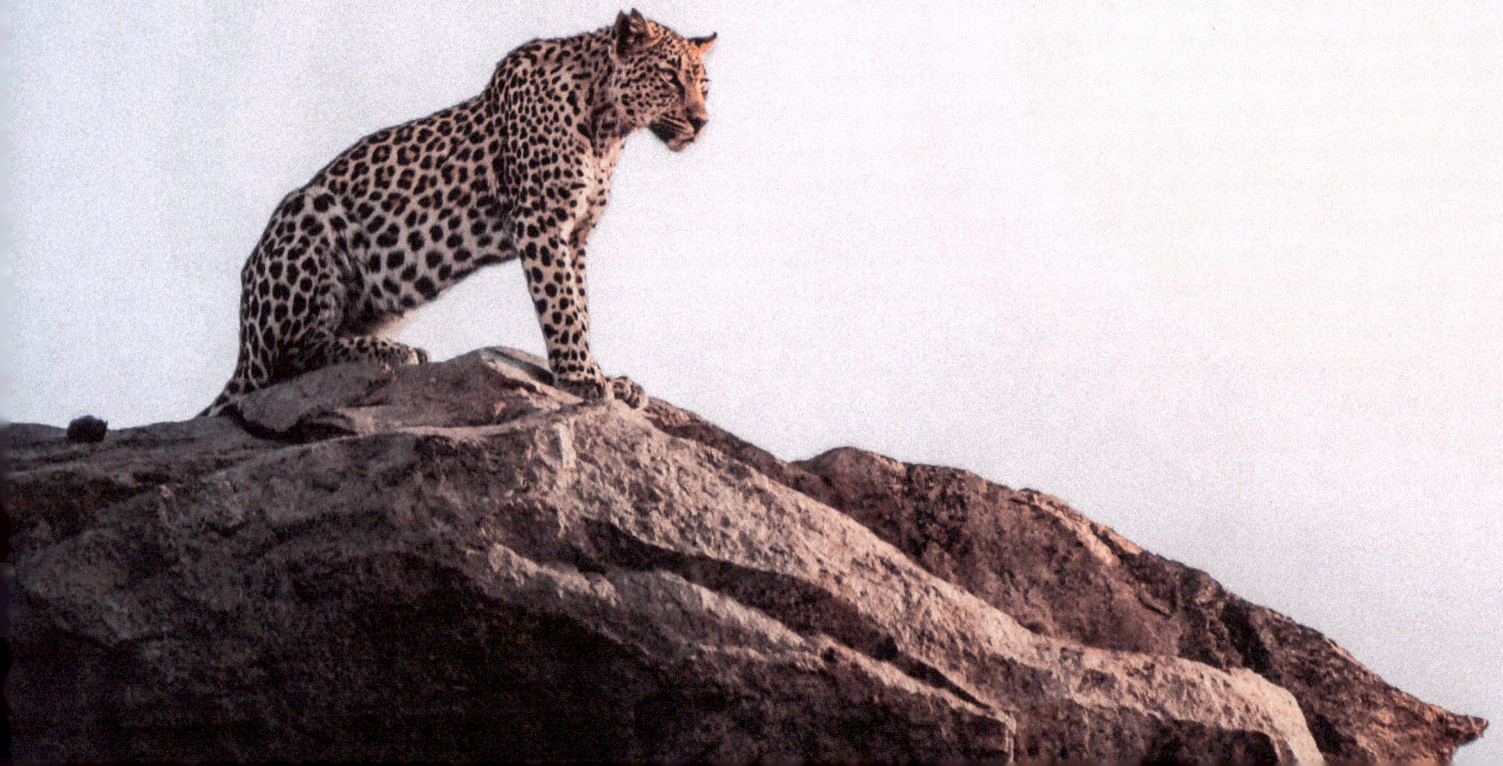

Understanding the mineral kingdom

The mineral kingdom is all about structure and organisation. The scientific characteristics are orderly and easily classified, for example, consider the periodic table and its formation. Issues associated with the mineral kingdom include factors such as formation, maintenance, and a loss of structure. Patients that possess similar characteristics are often logical people, who love stability and thrive within predictable environments. They are well organised, and this can often be reflected in the clothes they wear – either completely plain or symmetrical striped or orderly patterned attire. They enjoy structured thinking processes and choose occupations that demand these attributes, often becoming an engineer, accountant, business manager. They are high performers, achieving in their chosen industry, from parental care to global CEOs, these same characteristics of order and efficiency will be apparent. Their common issues involve developing a sense of self-accomplishment and maintaining the stability of their structure. A lack of money, or loss of relationship, or a failure in performance are at the core of their problems.

Their fundamental characteristics are always reflected in human form as stability, capability, toughness, performance, and security.

Understanding the plant kingdom

The fundamental essence of a plant is sensitivity. It is living and flexible yet remains firmly rooted into the soil and incapable of moving. It requires incredible adaptability to the subtle changes within the environment around it to survive and grow, and therefore it has to be sensitive to nuances and changes, both subtle and extreme.

A patient requiring a remedy from the plant kingdom will be extremely sensitive to all the changes occurring in their internal and external environment. Their energy is similar to the energy of a plant; (i.e., of a sensitive nature, influenced by many things, always adapting and bending to them). They can be easily affected emotionally and express this through their body language, speech, tone and gestures, especially their hands, that will move in many directions as they communicate. Often, but not always, people expressing themselves through the plant kingdom will be healers or therapists or choose a career path that encourages natural expression of their deep and unique sensitivity.

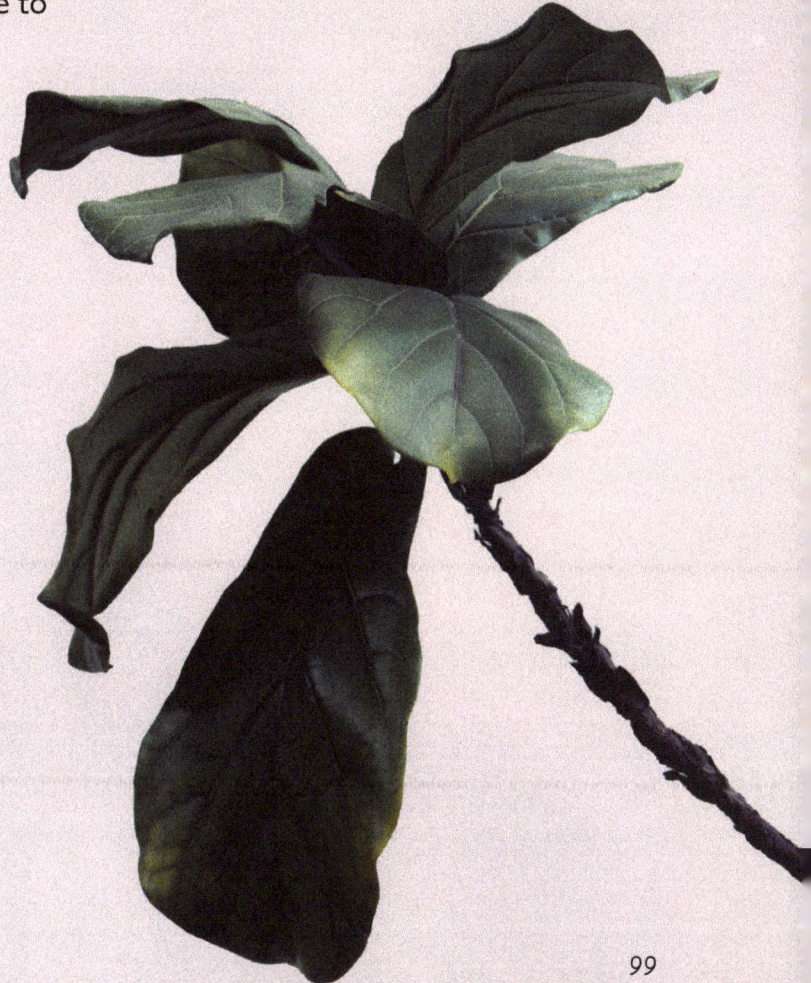

Folliculinum (Oestrone, follicular hormone)

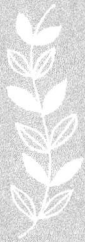

For some women, the oral contraceptive pill (OCP) doesn't agree with them and they suffer some side-effects. Some allopathic medications can leave an imprint on the nervous system, resulting in functional disturbances. When women have side effects during or when starting the OCP, there is a strong consideration that this is an obstacle to cure.

The OCP has a long list of side effects (including acne, which can be treated with the OCP, chloasma, vaginal thrush, headaches, and mood disturbances), which are important for me to consider when a patient presents with a seemingly unrelated illness.

The vaginal thrush with headaches and mood disturbance may be related to an increase in copper levels, which affect mood, sleep and liver function. Synthetic oestrogens will cause copper retention and biliary stasis in susceptible individuals. Many of these patients have low zinc.

When the copper is really high, zinc and vitamin C supplementation is beneficial. The folliculinum nosode is indicated here.

Folliculinum is made from ovarian follicle (folliculin), the natural hormone secreted by the ovaries and also known as estrogen.

The leading symptom for this remedy is control. Often the woman feels she is controlled by another. She is out of sorts with her rhythms. She is living out someone else's expectations. She loses her will. She overestimates her energy reserves. She is full of self-denial. She becomes a rescuer, addicted to rescuing people. She becomes drained. She has become a doormat. She has forgotten who she is and lacks individuality.

This remedy can be used for patients under extreme pressure who are not fully responding to homeopathy. These pressures could include:

⚡ Pressure from a personality or group on an individual, such as a dominant or possessive parent, friend or marriage partner, and where there is intolerant religious dominance.

⚡ Pressure of circumstance or work, such as that suffered by people who have worked to a point of exhaustion over time and seem to be incapable of recuperation or even responding to the indicated homeopathic medicine.

⚡ Pressure in adults from continued ill-health or slow recovery after recurrent or severe infection. This includes glandular fever or chronic fatigue syndrome. In these cases, carcinosinum can be used, but this can be followed up with folliculinum if the carc does not achieve a lasting response. The same applies to patients not responding after cortisone treatment.

Premenstrual symptoms

♈ Unable to tolerate noise, touch, or heat.

♈ Swollen breasts that are painful to touch.

♈ Panic attacks with huge mood swings.

♈ Very low or high libido.

♈ Nausea and vomiting.

♈ Prolonged and heavy bleeding with bright red blood and dark clots.

♈ Painful periods centred in the ovaries.

Clinical situations

♓ History of abuse, whether sexual, physical or psychological.

♓ Raynaud's disease.

♓ Eating disorders.

♓ Cardiovascular problems.

♓ Postnatal problems, difficulty bonding with the baby and children unable to separate from their mother.

Many women who were prescribed this remedy had symptoms between ovulation and menstruation. Women with these symptoms can be given folliculinum in 30 potency for several weeks. It is a powerful and deep-acting remedy that should not be taken without the professional guidance and supervision of a homeopath professionally trained and experienced in their use.

When you are testing deficiencies and identifying toxins, in addition to blood tests, a Hair Tissue Mineral Analysis (HTMA) can be used. It gives a wider perspective about mineral uptake and identifies the type and number of toxic elements which have been sequestered out of blood into tissue. Once the element arrives in tissue, it is usually not found in the blood. Blood reflects the current nutritional and toxic elements levels only, not past or accumulated exposure. Toxins in the body are exposed to stay in the blood for short periods, sometimes only days, until the body is able to remove them to other tissues, which is what we know as homeostasis.

Graphites (Black lead – plumbago)

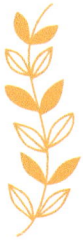

MATERIA MEDICA

Considered the antipsoric of great power, the graphite individual may present rather stout, of fair complexion, cold-blooded, with tendencies of skin problems such as cracking and lesions with a honey-like exudate. Constipation, frequent colds and swollen glands are also frequently seen. The female patient may have a delayed menstrual history.

This is mainly an antipsoric as well as an antipsychotic remedy.

Keynotes:

◊ Suited to women inclined to obesity, who suffer from habitual constipation and have a history of delayed menstruation.

◊ During menopause: excessive cautiousness, is timid and hesitates; is unable to decide about anything.

◊ Hard and cracked skin, especially the heels, palms and nipples.

◊ Fidgety when performing sedentary tasks, such as sitting at work.

◊ Eczema of eyelids; eruption is moist and fissured; lids are red and margins covered with scales or crusts.

◊ Sad, despondent; music makes them cry; they feel timid, fearsome, irresolute.

◊ Photophobia (fear of light).

◊ Acute sense of smell; can't stand flowers.

◊ Can be used for morning sickness during menstruation; very weak and prostrated.

◊ Sweats nauseate.

◊ Moist eruptions behind the ears.

They are better for darkness, wrapping up, open air, eating, and touch.

Aggravations are worse for fatty foods and sweets.

Ignatia amara
(St Ignatius bean or *Strychnos ignatia*)

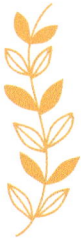

MATERIA MEDICA

Ignatia has traditionally been used for cases of hysteria and depression. Symptoms are related to emotional despair – such as shock, grief, hysterics, emotional and mental strain, and homesickness. The keynote for prescribing this remedy is grief.

This remedy is especially suited to nervous temperament; women of sensitive, easily excited nature, dark hair and skin but mild disposition; those who are quick to perceive and rapid in execution.

In striking contrast with the fair complexion, they are yielding and lachrymose, slow and indecisive.

The symptoms you may notice in this remedy are:

- Mentally, the emotional element is uppermost, and coordination of function is interfered with.
- Nervous temperament; women of sensitive, easily excited nature.
- Great contradictions. Sudden change in mental and physical states that oppose one another.
- Long sighs and yawning.
- Silently brooding; unhappy when in love; complaints come on after emotional trauma; changeable moods, hasty, apprehensive, easily frightened.
- Erratic, contradictory or spasmodic effects; often violent, with rigidity, twitching, tremors, spasms of single parts, cramps, jerks, twitches brought on by the mental state.
- Hyperesthesia of all senses, especially vision and hearing.
- Sensation of a lump in the throat, which is better for swallowing solids and indigestible foods; no thirst.
- Obstinate constipation; urging, pain; pain shoots high up in the rectum; prolapsed rectum, piles.

They are better for warmth (except the stomach is better for cold food and drink), being kept amused, profuse urination, and pressure.

There is a marked intolerance of cigarette smoke.

Sepia officinalis (Cuttlefish)

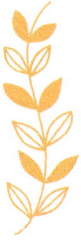

MATERIA MEDICA

This remedy has traditionally been given to tall, dark-haired, narrow-hipped women who have a history of menstrual disturbances and a tendency to prolapse, especially of the abdominal organs. Adapted to persons of a rigid fibre, but mild and easy disposition. Their faces are pale, sallow and yellowish with sagging and heavy eyelids and they frequently experience outbreaks of herpes around the lips, behind the ears, and on the back of the neck.

It acts especially on the portal system, with venous congestion.

Keynotes:

- Commonly complaining of 'bearing down' sensation and 'ball' sensation in their parts.
- Indolent; averse to exertion.
- Weakness.
- Hypersensitive to noise and bright lights.
- Loathes fat and milk, craves acids and sour foods.
- Diarrhoea from boiled milk.
- Itching and burning which is not relieved by scratching.
- Sluggish, cold extremities, cold in spots.
- Yellow complexion.
- Bearing down sensation, especially in women, upon whose organism it has the most pronounced effect.
- Chills easily; lack of vital heat, especially in chronic disease.
- A marked aversion to company when they are unwell.
- They are utterly exhausted and may cry when telling their symptoms.
- Irritable, domineering, can't stand opposition; absence of joy; indifferent to family due to exhaustion.
- Irritability due to tiredness, wants to be left alone.
- Herpes; ringworm.
- Aching in the lumbar region, better for hard pressure in back.
- Nausea at the sight or smell of food or a gnawing hunger.
- Obstinate constipation, especially during pregnancy, and even with a soft stool.

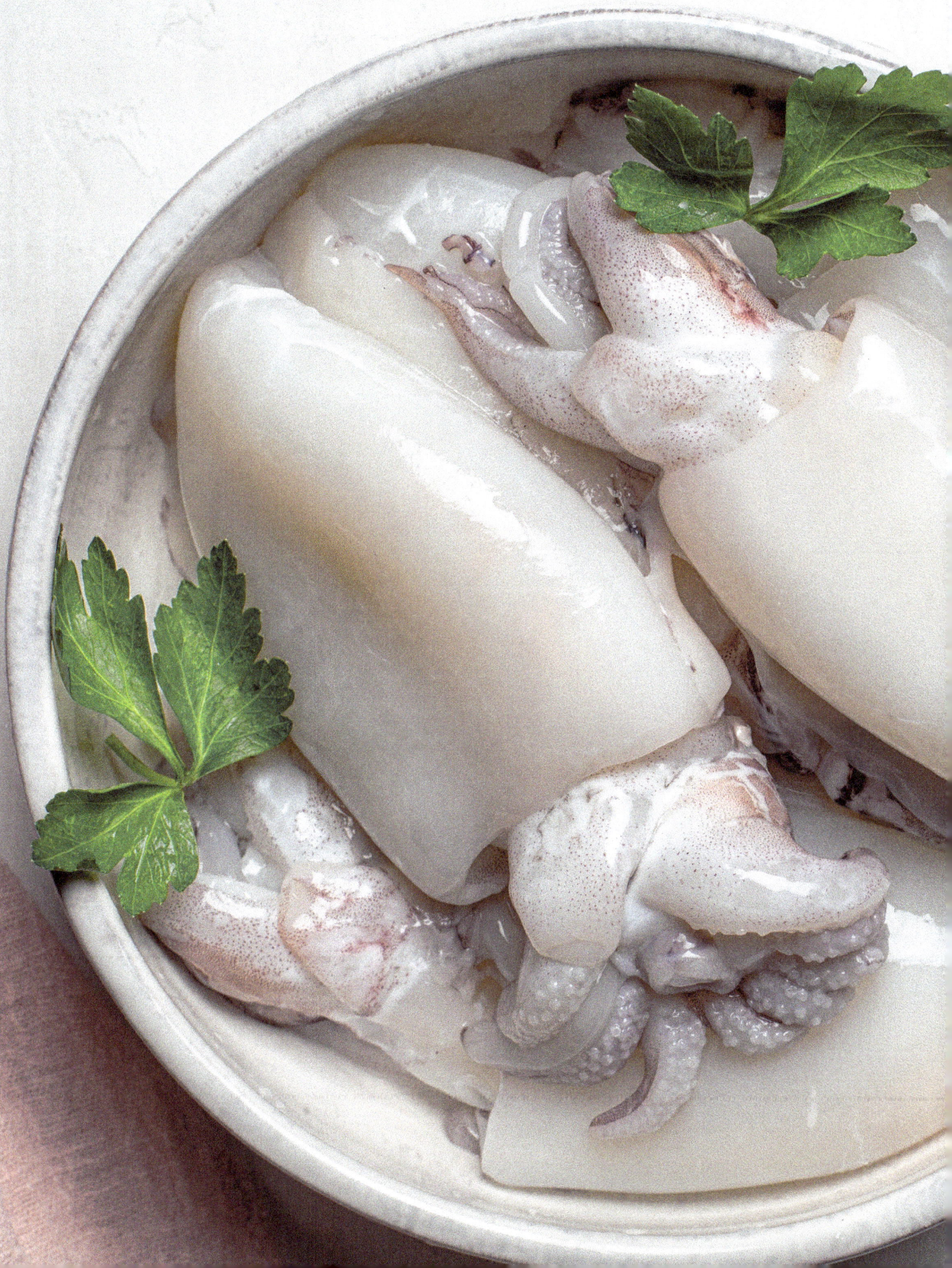

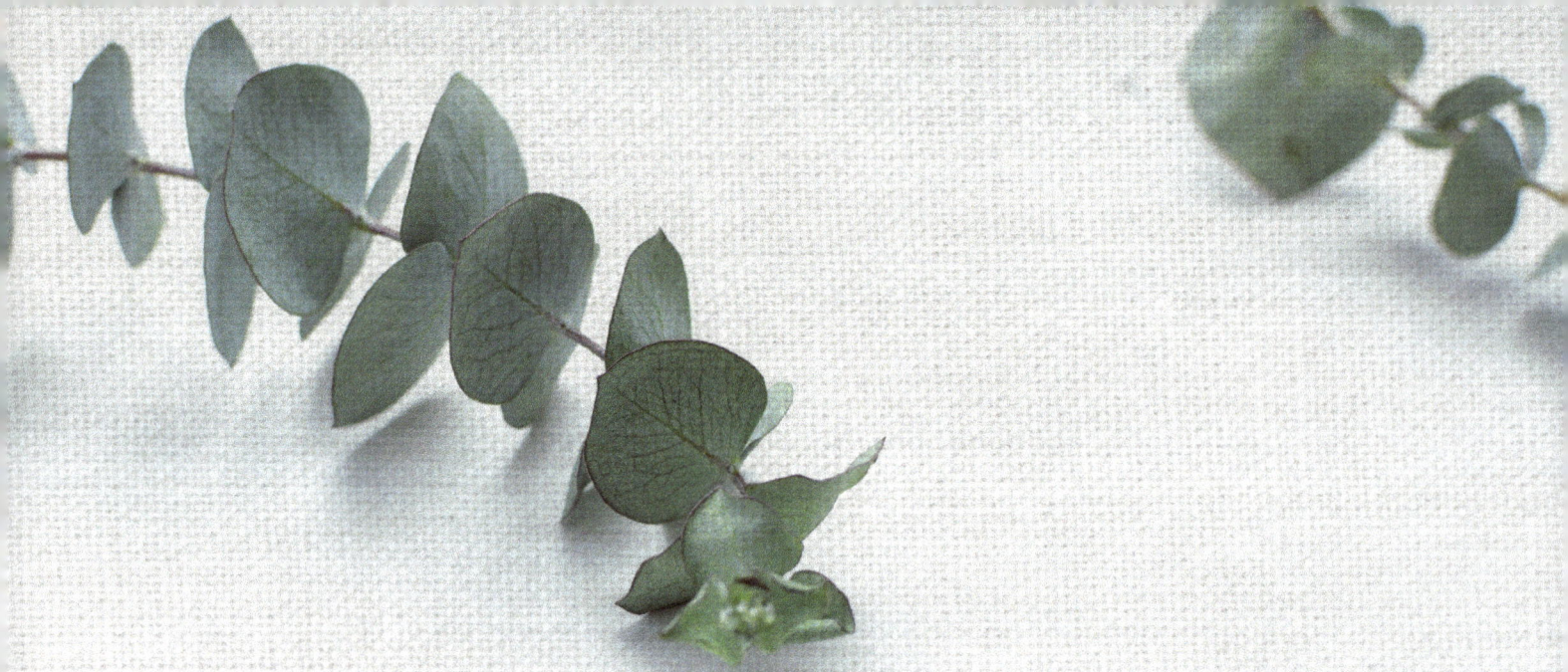

Homeopathy works
with your body;
we're not adding
anything here.

Zincum metallicum (Zinc)

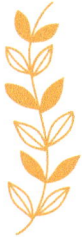

The homeopathic remedy zincum is used for treating a zinc absorption condition, among other conditions. This metal seems to act principally upon the nervous system. Burt says that "What iron is to the blood, zinc is to the nerves".

Case study notes:

- 40-year-old female.

- Dietary intake is adequate.

- No history of recurrent virus infections.

- No current skin disease present.

- Severe zinc deficiency shown on recent OligoScan report.

- Past history of zinc deficiency.

- Responded well to homeopathic treatment in the past.

In this case, the patient's symptoms tell me that zinc supplementation is not the best mode of action for her zinc deficiency, as it is not associated with a lack of nutrients, but the disposition to not absorb and retain zinc.

Zincum is useful here and a triple split dose (TSD) given in a very low potency, one week before administering the constitutional remedy. This has traditionally been used to remove the blocks the body had towards absorption and retention of this crucial nutrient. As with other minerals, zinc deficiency is often an obstacle to cure.

Other indicated uses for Zincum Met include:

- The nervous system is of most importance.

- Convulsive twitching and fidgety feet are the guiding symptoms.

- Brain fog covers a large part of the zinc action.

- Tissues are worn out faster than they can be repaired.

- Coryza; spasmodic cough; asthmatic bronchitis; constriction and cutting in chest.

- Melancholia.

- Palpitation, and palpitation with anxiety.

- Spasmodic movement of the heart.

- Very sensitive to noise.

- Vertigo.

- Heartburn after sweet foods.

- Defective vitality.

- Grinding of teeth.

HOMEOPATHY AND COLOURS

Some practitioners will use colour preferences as a homeopathic symptom. Homeopathic colour diagnoses (colour preferences and aversions) have been clinically identified and become a valuable addition to the *Materia Medica*. The colour repertory, *Colours in Homeopathy*, is in worldwide use and is now available in five languages.

Some homeopaths will ask the patient to choose a colour from a provided colour chart. Choosing a particular colour indicates a symptom that relates to a certain remedy.

When prescribing this way, it can be a useful tool to come to a conclusion with a prescription for a patient. It is not used by every homeopath, nor in every consultation by homeopaths who do use it, and it definitely should not be used as a substitute for *Materia Medica*.

The natural colour choice selected by the patient is a prime indicator in the selection of the practitioner's prescription of a remedy, and is a good therapeutic tool.

Many patients can also have a definite aversion to a certain colour, but this has been less frequently worked with because the preference is easier to assess.

Using colour preference can be seamlessly implemented into the typical homeopathic process but should not act as a substitute or replacement for best practice. It can certainly help identify the patient's dispositional symptoms but is not thorough enough to formulate a prescription, or detour from the foundational works of *Materia Medica*. The homeopath's experience and knowledge of *Materia Medica* is vital, as any and all prescribed remedies must be similar to the disease picture and disposition.

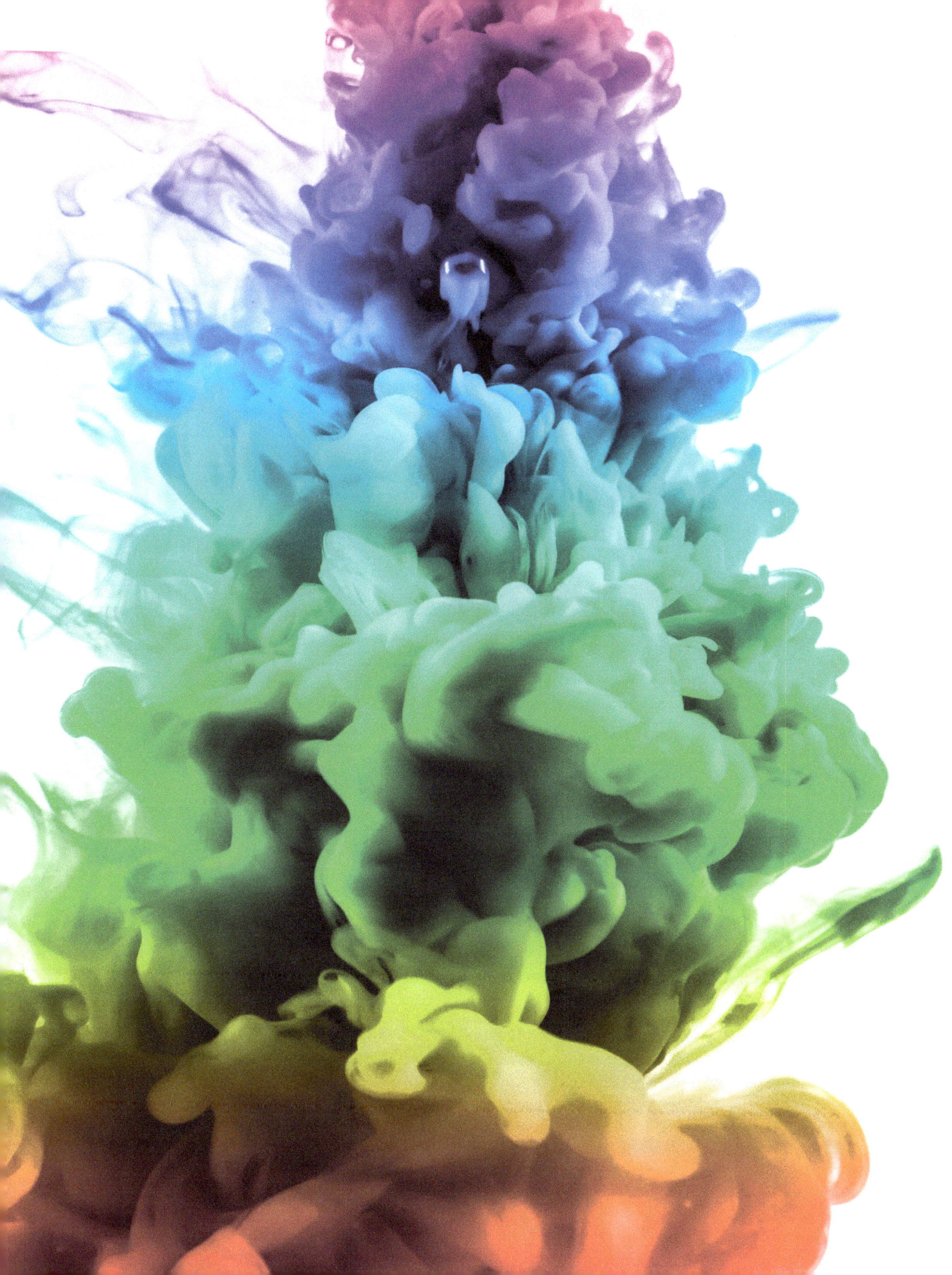

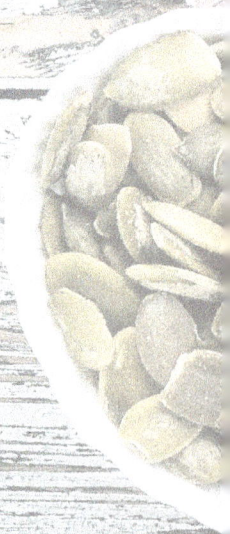

NUTRITION

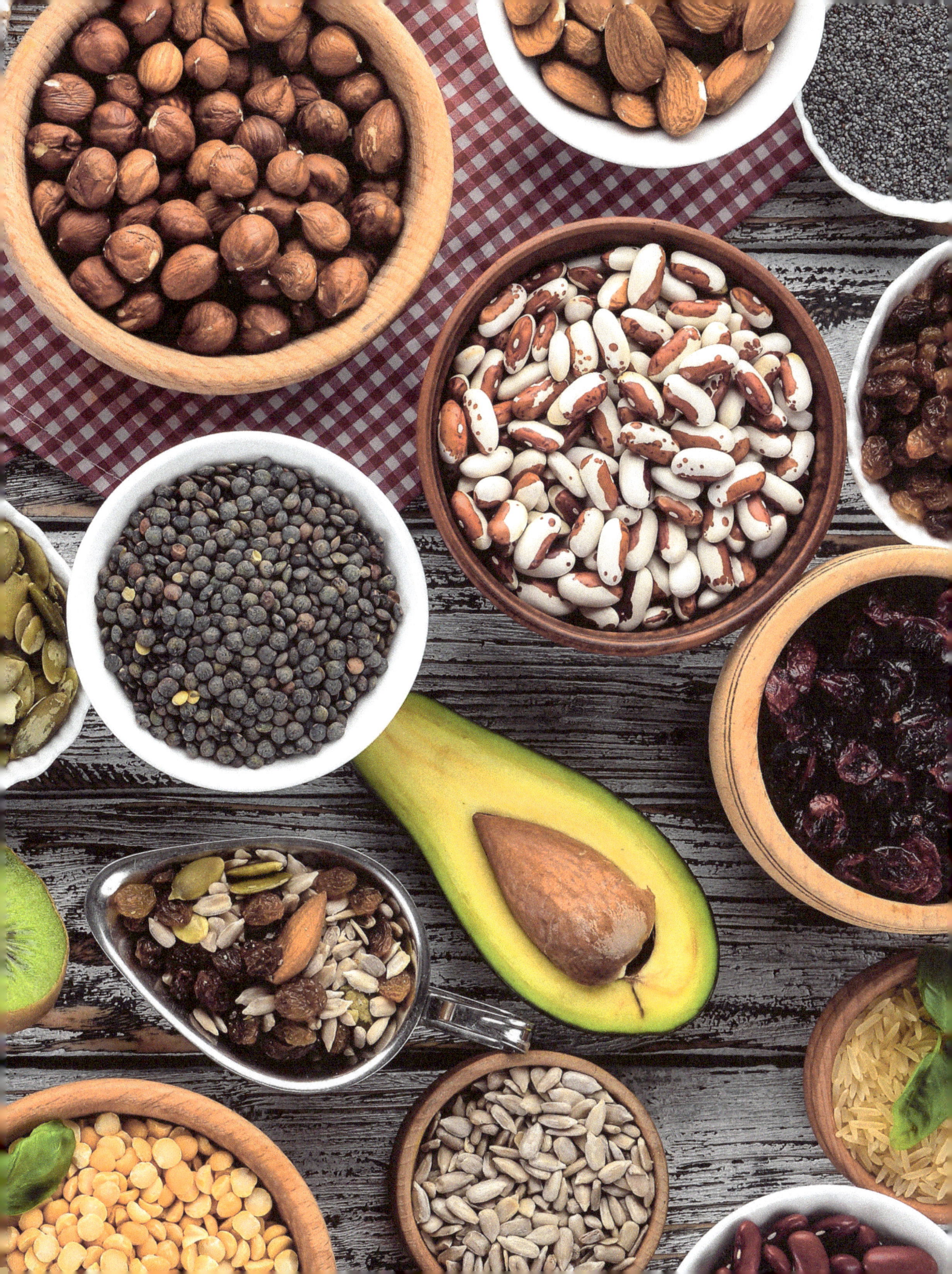

Homeopathy is a highly individualised system of medicine that can help with nutrition, which also requires an individual approach. Nutritional deficiency is an easily overlooked and common obstacle to cure.

A homeopath is well-informed of the conditions that specific nutritional deficiencies can cause. When seeing a patient, the homeopath will check appetite and diet, giving them vital information about personal preferences that they incorporate into the prescription and nutritional deficiencies.

Homeopathic medicine has the capacity to enhance mineral absorption, but it is unlikely to be a substitute for frank deficiency. It is a system that gently stimulates the body's energy flow back to equilibrium, allowing the body to do what it does best – heal itself.

Everything you consume either fights disease or feeds it.

Food as medicine

Nutrition is a highly individualised subject, just as homeopathy is a highly individualised system. The needs of the body vary during different stages of life and each patient must find their most comfortable and beneficial diet. We are not only what we eat, we are also how well we digest and absorb our food.

Fresh food is great – freshly picked fruits and vegetables that are in season, rather than frozen or packaged varieties, are best. Organic produce is also a great option.

Gut health is imperative for many functions of the body. Gut bugs help regulate metabolism and nutrient absorption. It is a complex system that is very important to our overall health.

Obstacles to cure

Aphorism: "The careful investigation into obstacles to cure is so much more necessary in the case of patients affected by chronic disease, as their diseases are usually aggravated by such noxious influences and other disease-causing errors in the diet and regimen, which often pass unnoticed." – Samuel Hahnemann

Some medications will disrupt the microbial actions in your gut, either by preventing and slowing bacterial growth or killing them. For example, antibiotics will predispose an individual to gut dysbiosis.

Corticosteroids are a common prescription in conventional medicine for inflammatory conditions. The prolonged use of corticosteroids depletes mineral absorption, particularly calcium, leading to osteoporosis. Some useful natural anti-inflammatories are turmeric, boswellia and glucosamine (which is used to repair joints and reduce pain).

Sugar is often an obstacle to cure. This might be really obvious, but I can't tell you how many people easily dismiss it. The link between sugar and inflammation is convincingly high. Patients whose presenting complaints are acne, arthritis, fibromyalgia or other general inflammatory diseases should avoid sugar (including cough syrups). Sugar prevents the proper function of the immune system. With a compromised immune system, the skin remains an eliminating organ for toxic waste.

Gluten are the proteins found in wheat, rye and barley; these cannot be eaten by people with coeliac disease. These proteins create a leaky gut. A leaky gut allows gluten and many other foreign toxic substances to penetrate the body. They need to be eliminated and the skin is one of the acting organs for elimination. An option I have advised some patients is to start by eliminating gluten from the diet.

If after doing this, there is no change in their skin, I don't think their efforts have gone unnoticed (not internally anyway), as usually their general health and long-term prognosis has likely improved. This means the deeper imbalance has been brought to the forefront, and the body is now showing signs and symptoms relating to the patient holistically, and not created artificially by the gluten that was creating unhealthy symptoms for them. Now with this clean slate we have a clear picture and can proceed with more accurate treatment from a modality like homeopathy, and appropriately prescribed remedies. Watch as the magic unfolds!

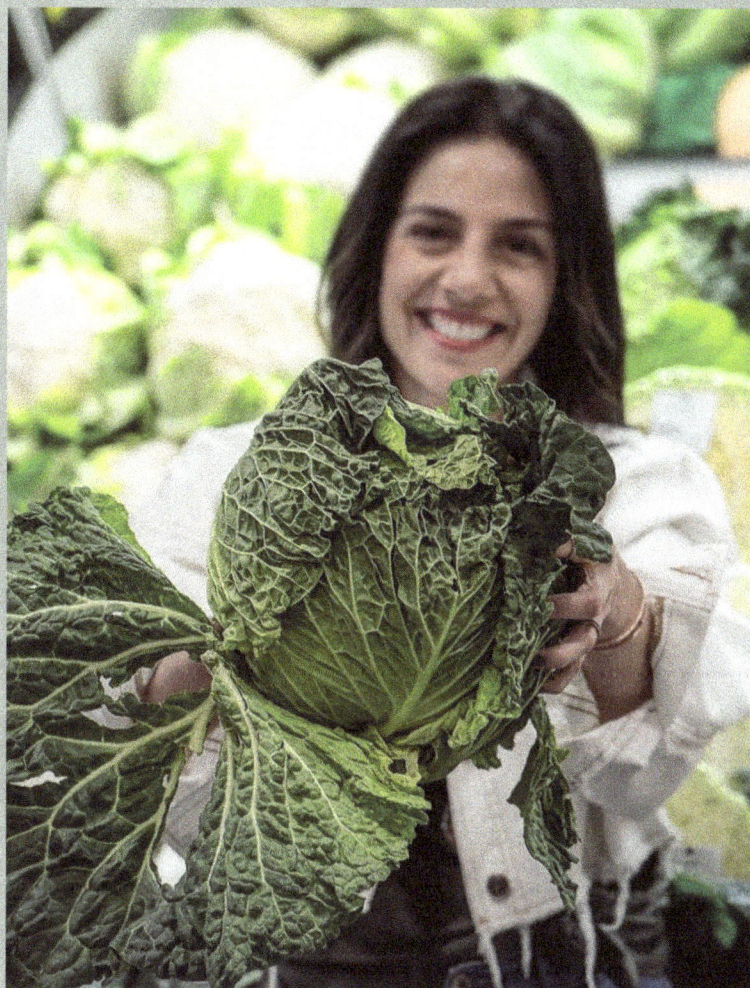

Zinc

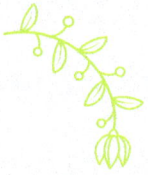

The functions of the body that critically rely on the mineral zinc include: normal growth and development, immune function, skin health, appetite regulation, and endocrine function. It is essential for the normal function of multiple body enzymes and known for killing some viruses on contact.

Zinc deficiency is most easily recognisable through looking for white spots on the fingernails, and testing zinc levels will also show zinc deficiency. If you constantly get viruses and you are unresponsive or relapse after homeopathic treatment, then I would suspect a zinc deficiency and recommend a zinc taste test or HTMA (Hair Tissue Mineral Analysis).

As with other mineral deficiencies, zinc deficiency is often an obstacle to cure. However, supplementation should be monitored, as excess zinc can predispose to bacterial infections due to it creating copper deficiency. It should not be self-prescribed.

Generally for zinc absorption, we need sufficient levels of vitamin B6 and magnesium. When treating nutritionally I suggest a renowned quality supplement as they will contain both of these. However, as described in the homeopathic remedies chapter of this book, the homeopathic remedy *Zincum Metallicum* is used for treating zinc absorption conditions. In addition, as mentioned, prescribing constitutionally is another beneficial way of treating holistically because once the baseline is stable I expect vitamin and mineral levels to improve as well.

Some symptoms of zinc deficiency include:

· Disturbed sleep

· Loss of smell and taste

· Poor concentration

· Poor wound healing

· Stretch marks

· Premenstrual syndrome

· Repeated viral, yeast and fungal infections resulting from poor immunity

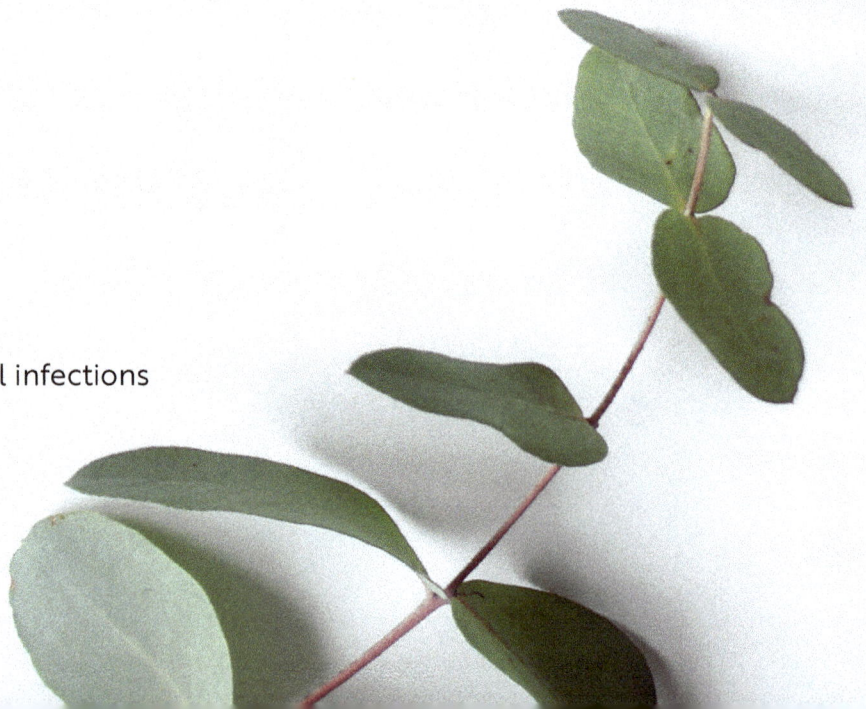

The natural healing force within each of us is the greatest force in getting well.
HIPPOCRATES

Some diseases associated with zinc deficiency include:

- Acne

- Dermatitis

- Psoriasis

- Autism

- Heavy metal accumulation

- Infertility

- Depression

- Rheumatoid arthritis

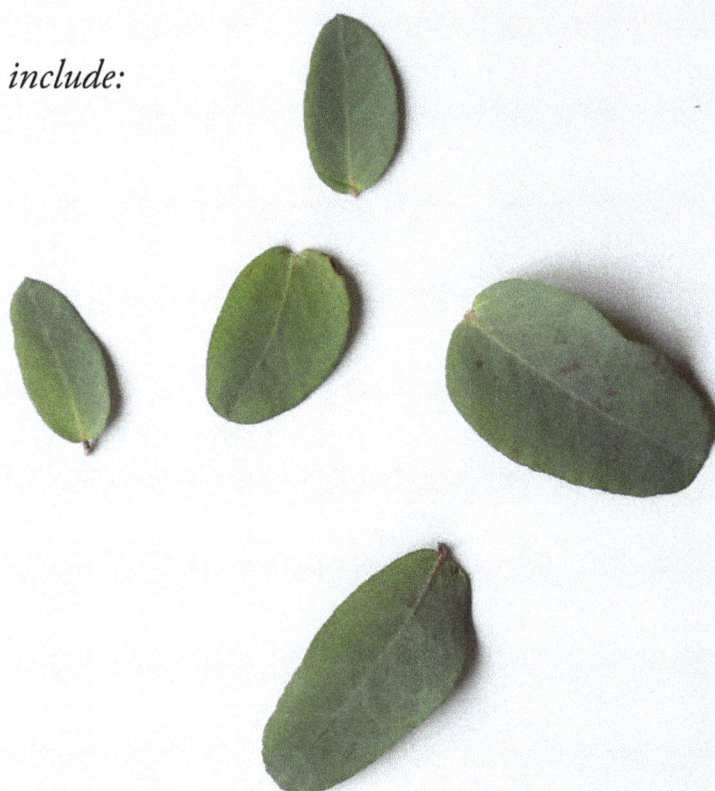

Causes of zinc deficiency include:

- High alcohol intake

- Excess copper

- Foods grown in zinc-deficient soils

- A high-grain diet, which blocks zinc absorption

- Medications such as cortisone, diuretics and anti-inflammatories

- Poor diet (including poor vegetarian or vegan diets)

- Stress

Sugar

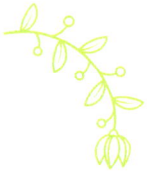

People are often so particular with every detail of their life, from cars to homes to clothes, but they cut corners when it comes to their health, and the food and medicines they consume.

Looking at your nutrition means dealing with the most neglected obstacle to cure and ensuring sustainable health. For example, let's talk about sugar.

Carbohydrates, when broken down or converted into glucose, fuel the body and the brain. However, excessive intake of sugar via processed foods and sweetened beverages may lead to overeating, which can contribute to obesity, diabetes, and cardiovascular disease.

Sugar prevents the proper function of the immune system. With a compromised immune system, the skin remains the eliminating organ for toxic waste. It won't matter how expensive your cosmetic products or treatments are, because they won't deliver sustainable results.

Your health is your wealth. It's a lifestyle choice, and cheap costs the most! Look within.

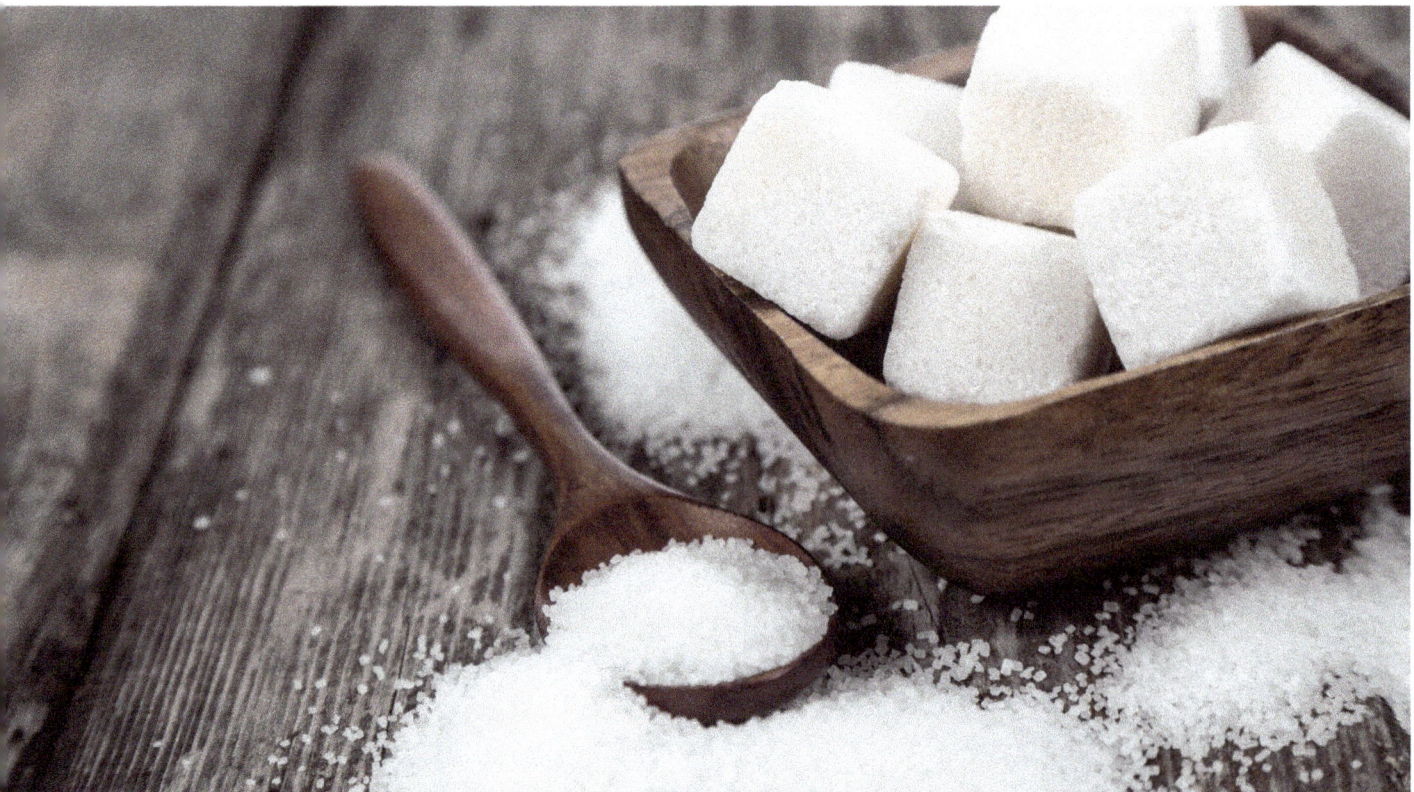

It's a lifestyle choice.

Ginger

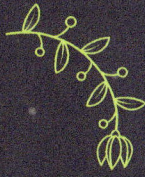

Ginger helps to stimulate the heart and contributes to heart health. It is also known for its role in reducing the inflammatory response.

I will often cut some fresh ginger root, add boiling water to it and sip on it as a tea; you can also buy ginger tea. It gives a soothing and calming effect. It's also good for indigestion, nausea, cold and flu symptoms and sore throats.

Cardamom and turmeric are also members of the ginger family.

Cardamom has traditionally been used to relieve stomach upsets and heartburn. Chewing cardamom seeds is known to be an effective breath freshener; it sweetens the breath in a similar way to gum or mints.

Turmeric is considered an anti-inflammatory herb and can be used to reduce the risk of gallstones. It can also be used with barley and yogurt for sunburn relief. To use this remedy, you should mix equal parts turmeric, barley, and yogurt, and apply to the sunburned area.

Tip: I often enjoy a pear and ginger smoothie. Pear is one of the only fruits with little to zero sugar (which is very beneficial for diabetics), and with ginger's mighty medicinal properties, it is a staple in my kitchen and my number one spice heading into winter.

Zingiber Officinalis (also called 'zing') is a homeopathic remedy made from ginger. This remedy reflects states of debility in the digestive tract, sexual system, and respiratory system. It has also been used in cases of kidney disease.

The respiratory features of zing include: hoarseness, smarting below the larynx, difficulty breathing, and a dry hacking cough.

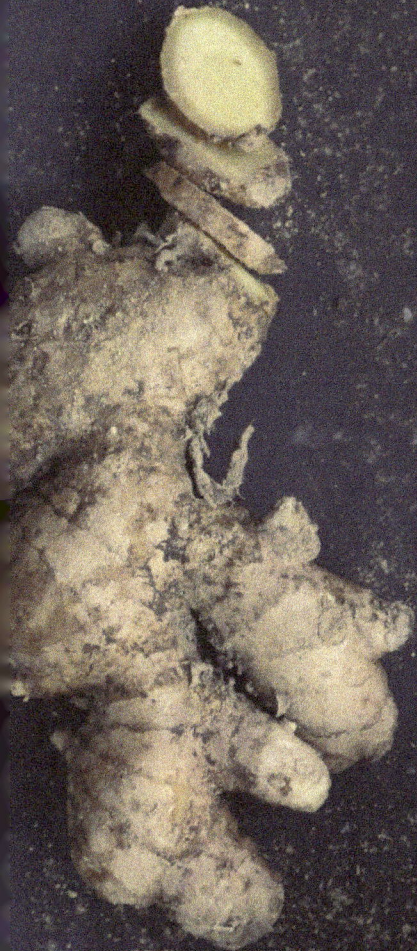

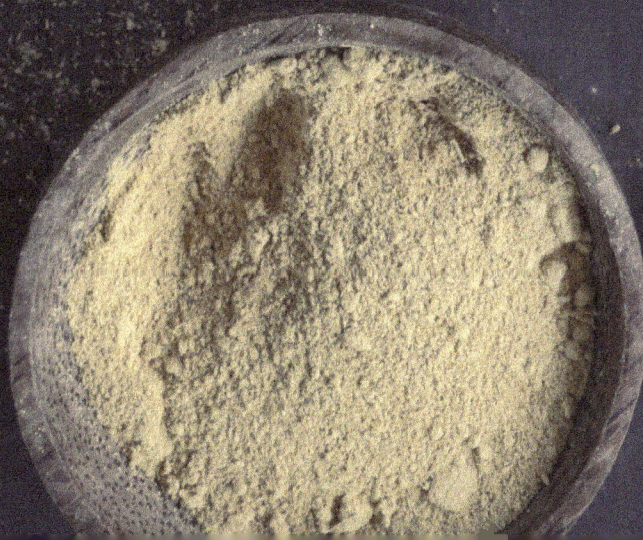

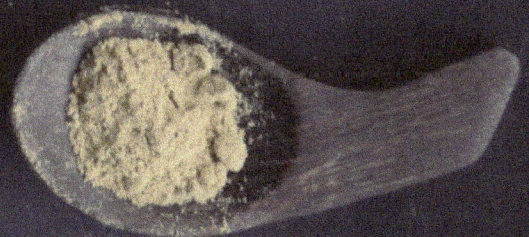

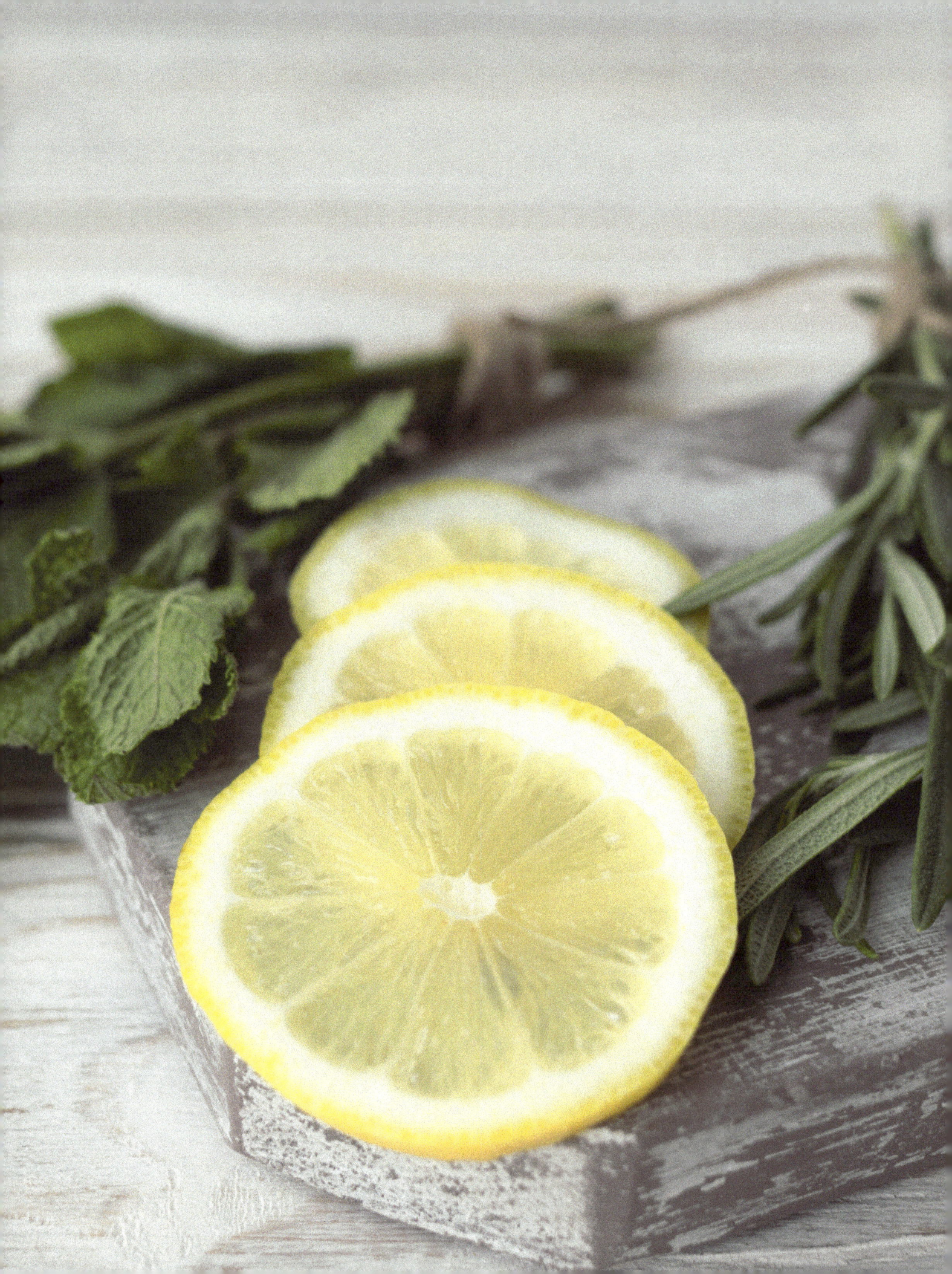

Lemons

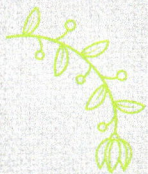

Lemons have many uses:

- Can help heal a hoarse voice, inflammation of the mouth and throat, and complaints of the digestive system.

- Useful for weight control, gout and urine retention, boosting immunity and energy levels.

- A useful remedy for asthma – fresh lemon slices or wedges can be very beneficial when taken in the morning, in a glass of warm water.

- Useful for insomnia, nervousness, and heart palpitations.

- Is a powerful natural cleaner, helping keep our insides – stomach, liver and intestines – in good condition, and preventing kidney stones.

- A useful remedy for arthritis and vitamin C deficiency. Vitamin C is needed to produce collagen, which strengthens the capillaries that supply the skin.

- Vitamin C enhances absorption of nonheme iron from foods consumed concurrently.

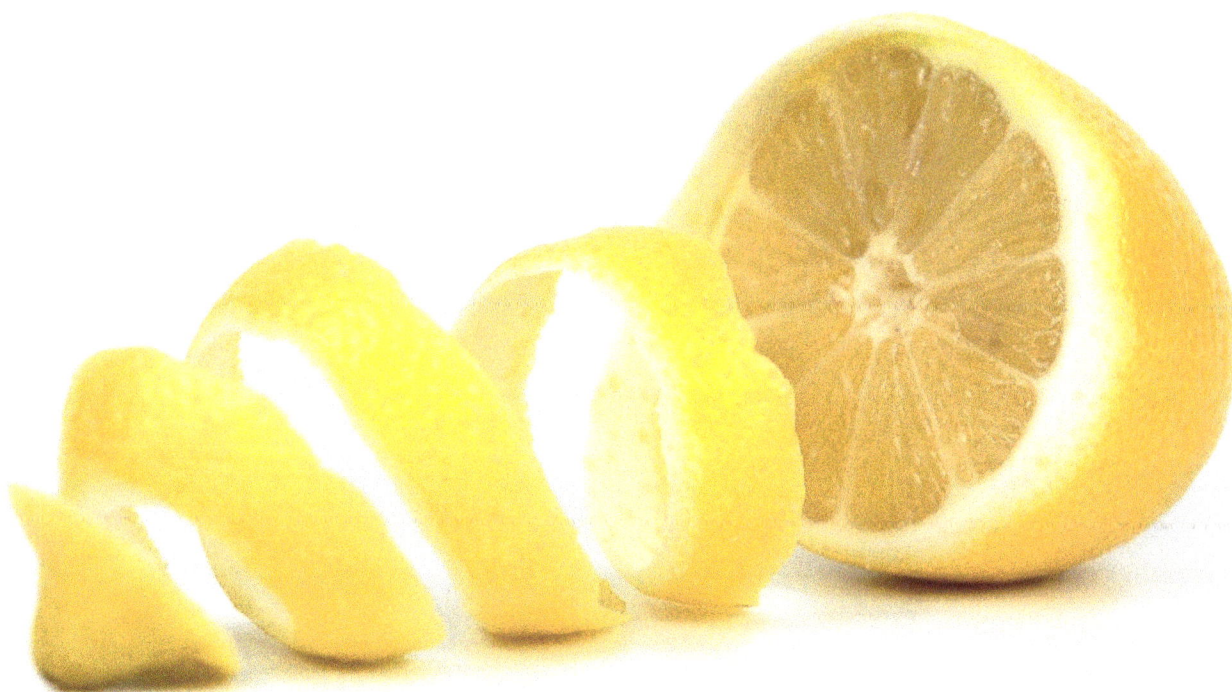

Coconut

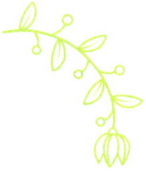

There are oodles of health benefits from this wonder fruit. Strictly speaking, a coconut is a drupe, but it can also be referred to as a fruit, nut, or seed.

Here are just a few of my favourite uses:

· Can be used for its water, milk, oil and meat.

· It's a healthy fat.

· Can be consumed and used externally.

· Strengthens the immune system and the body's defences.

· The oil can be used to cook safely at high temperatures.

· Research says coconut oil actually protects the heart from disease.

· Supports thyroid function.

· Lowers cholesterol.

· It's antimicrobial and has been shown to destroy invading pathogens.

· Helps weight loss because of the way the oil is digested, by raising our metabolic rate and stimulating the liver into action; you'll probably feel more full as well.

· Skin and hair repair – coconut definitely beats those pricey hair and beauty products. It gave me the shiniest hair I've ever had, and it is a beautiful moisturiser to keep your skin hydrated and youthful.

· My personal favourite: coconut water aids exercise recovery, restores hydration and replenishes electrolytes lost during exercise. I started drinking coconut water approximately eight years ago when I started training regularly and the energy boosts were incredible!

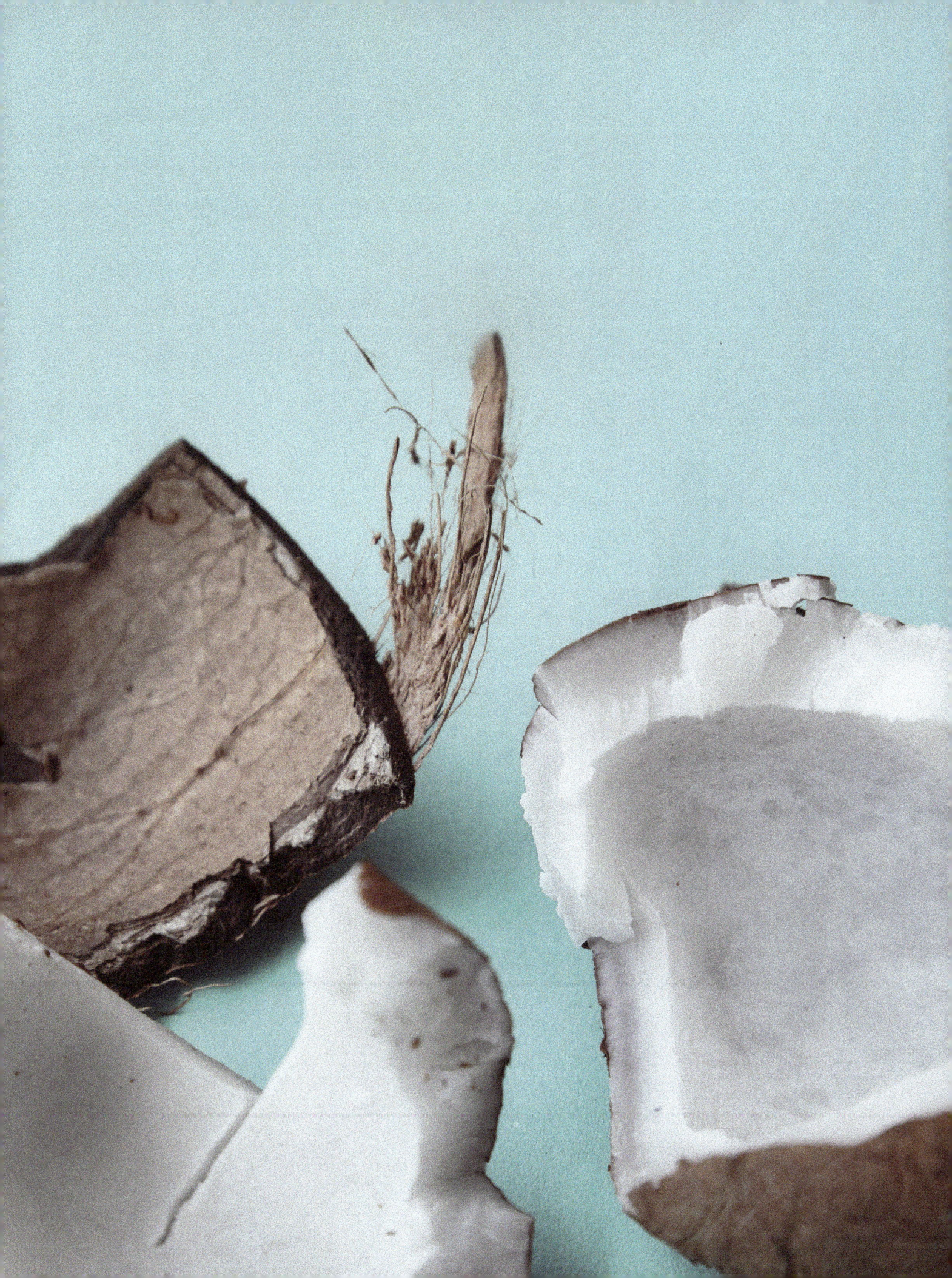

YOUR FOOD IS YOUR MOOD

The energy- and mood-enhancing effects of a diet enriched with multicoloured organic whole foods are priceless. When you eat a wide range of produce that varies in colour, you introduce different phytonutrients into your diet, which provide multiple health benefits, including improved mood.

The intimate connection between gut and brain can be linked to numerous conditions including anxiety, stress, diverticulitis and depression. When your gut microbiota is unbalanced, your mental state can suffer.

Health comes from the inside-out!

Gut health as a gateway to better brain function

Serotonin, often referred to as the 'happy' chemical, is a chemical in the brain that contributes to wellbeing and happiness. A vast majority of serotonin is produced in the gut, not the brain, so when you're taking pleasure from love and connection with friends and family, you're actually indirectly improving your gut health.

Exercise and massage are two simple ways of increasing serotonin naturally, and taking care of your gut will also help boost this wonderful chemical.

The vagus nerve

The vagus is a large nerve that communicates involuntary functions, such as heart rate and immune response, from the brain to the body. It plays a major part in the digestive process, directing stomach muscles to contract in order to move food through the digestive tract.

Just as a leaky gut plays a role in brain function, poor brain health, brain trauma or brain degeneration contribute to a leaky gut by decreasing activation of the vagus nerve. Low vagal tone can impede gut function and contribute to digestive disorders. The vagus nerve also provides a communication pathway between the brain and gut bacteria, and could influence microbiota composition, either positively or negatively.

Parasites and leaky gut

It is possible to unknowingly host a variety of parasites, including pinworms, roundworms or tapeworms, in the gut. Nature has several botanicals that work to provide natural support to help the body expel parasites, and they also have antioxidant properties that support the anti-inflammatory response.

Oregano extract has been used for the management of gastrointestinal infections in natural medicine for decades. Oregano extract is said to assist with the elimination of parasites and stimulate lymphocyte production, enhancing the body's immune system.

Olive leaf extract contains compounds that have extremely potent antioxidant, anti-inflammatory and immune-supporting properties. It serves as a natural agent with antifungal, antimicrobial, antiviral and antiparasitic properties. They also display antipathogenic effects, including inhibiting pathogenic organism reproduction.

As the adage says ...

I'm more interested in
what type of person has
a disease than what type
of disease a person has.

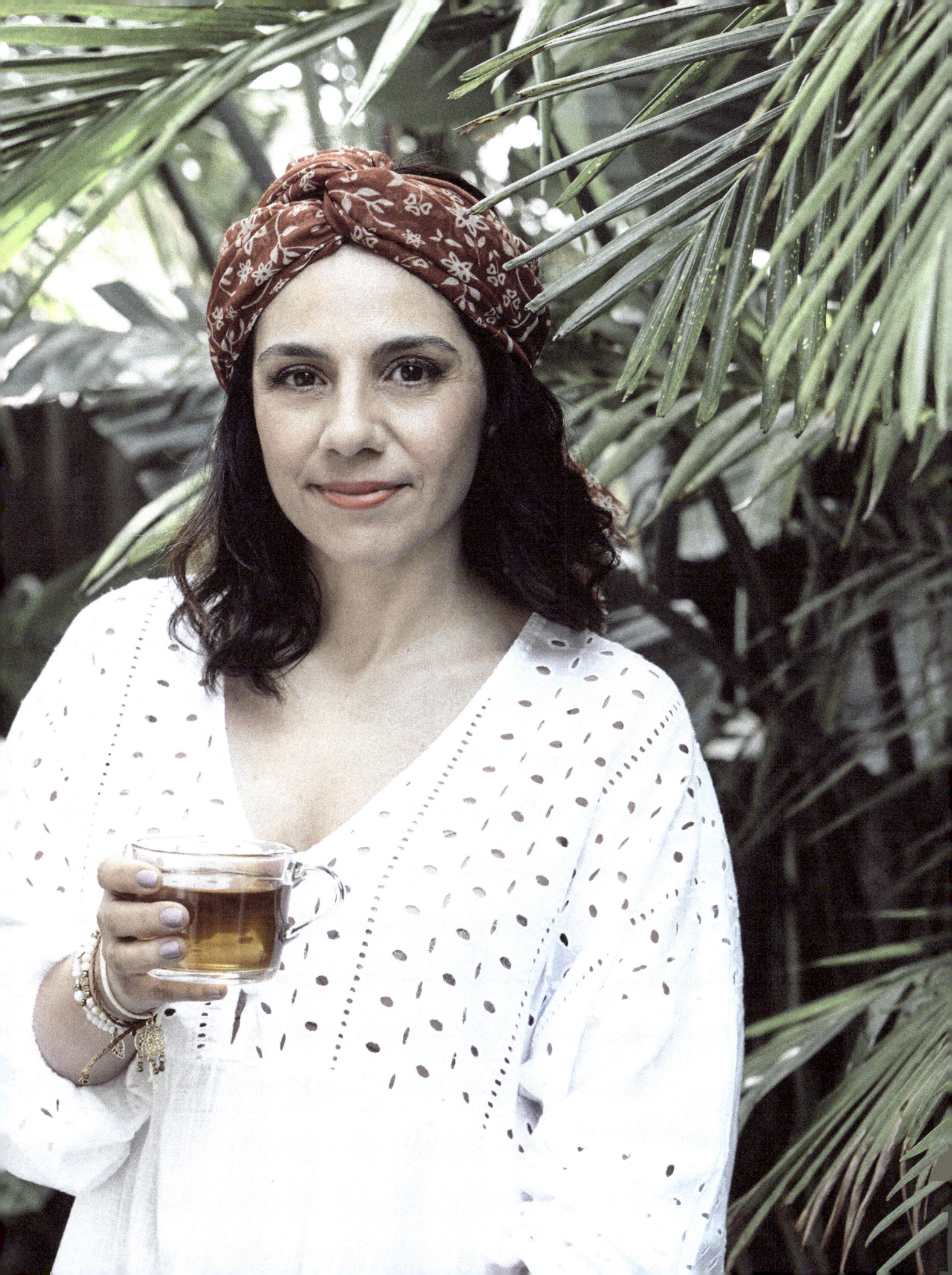

Grapefruit

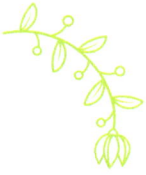

There are huge health benefits from the grapefruit. Drinking chilled grapefruit juice, and particularly during winter, will increase your vitamin C absorption. Grapefruit has many benefits from its nutrients, vitamins, potassium and lycopene. Vitamin A boosts the immune system; potassium lowers blood pressure, and lycopene could reduce the risk of developing some cancers. Grapefruit also contains calcium, sugar and phosphorus.

Grapefruit is contraindicated with some medications, so as always, check with your healthcare provider before consuming it.

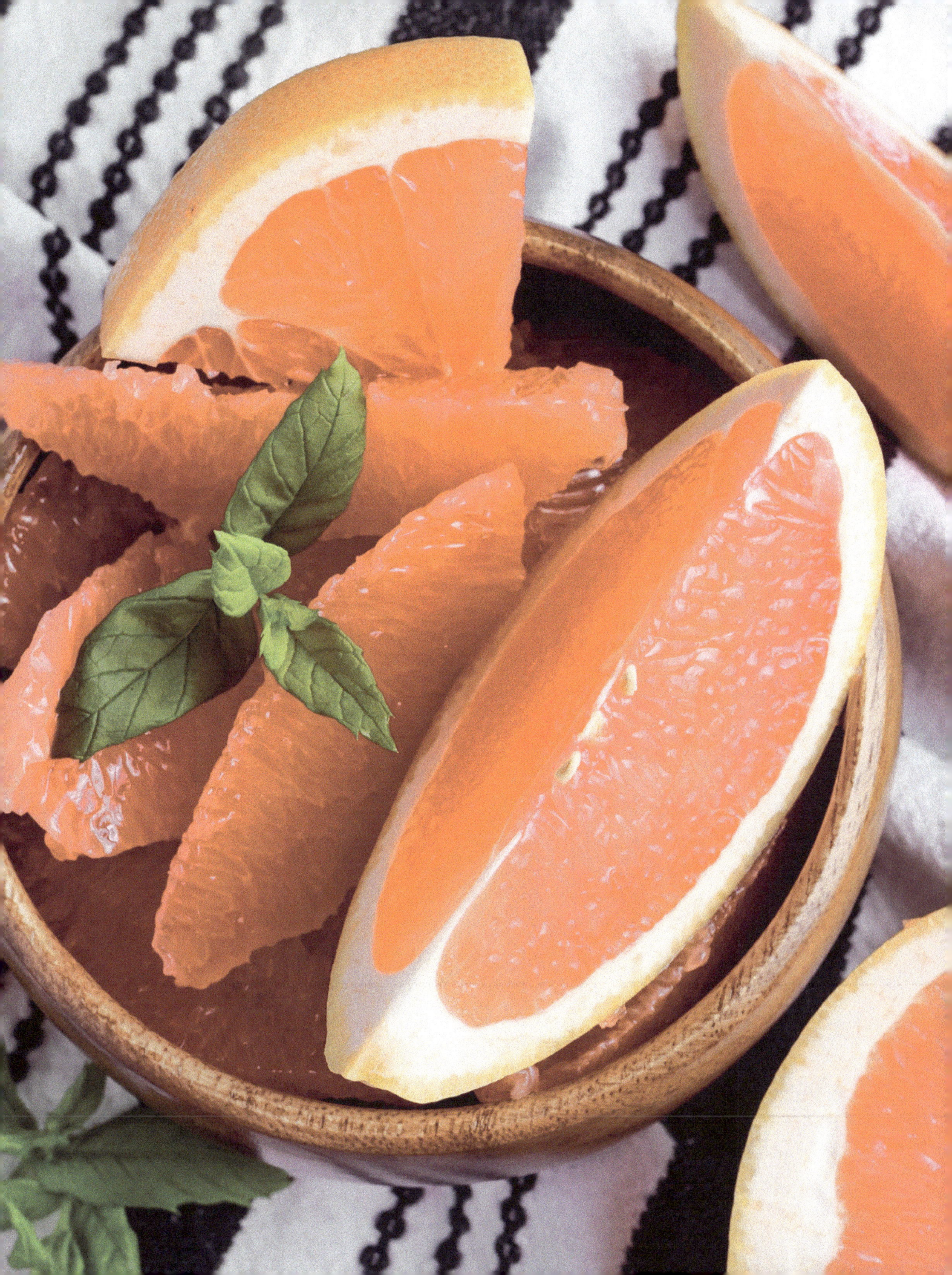

Garlic

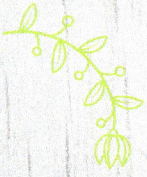

Garlic is a nutritional powerhouse. This natural antibacterial is thought to help prevent ailments including heart disease, stroke and hypertension. Garlic has been used as medicine for thousands of years, helping to fight off infection and support the immune system.

Handy hint: Garlic can help warts! Try cutting a piece of fresh garlic and putting it on your wart. Cover it with a Band-Aid and wait 24 hours. Repeat if necessary.

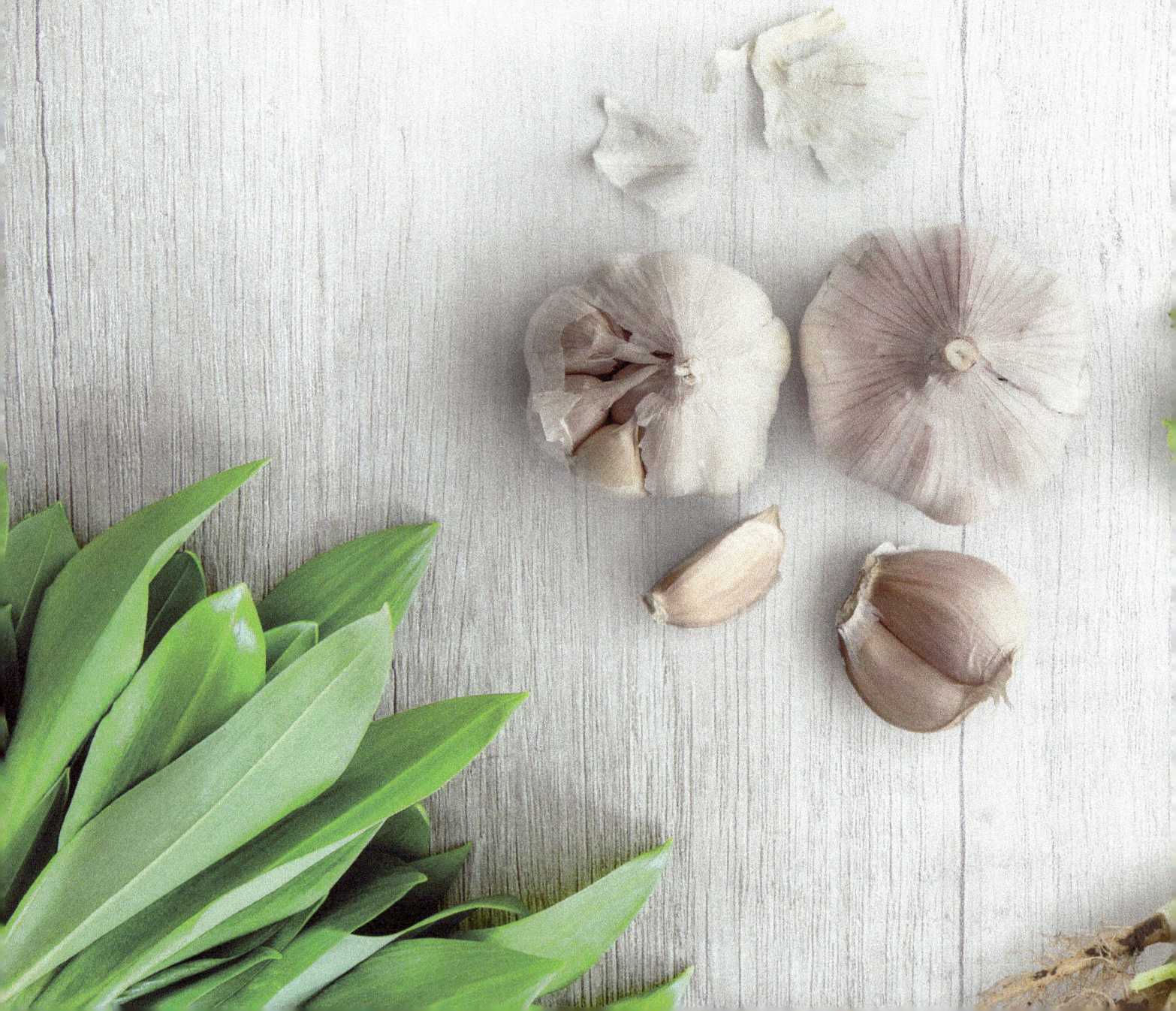

Lettuce

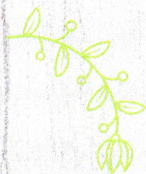

When you plant a seed for fruit, veggies or herbs to grow, you need the right environment for it to thrive – and the same principle applies to our health. Viruses, bacteria and disease need a favourable environment to take up residency in your body.

Tip: My favourite nutritional health benefits of lettuce include anti-inflammatory, antibacterial and antifungal properties. Its array of vitamins, minerals, and other bioactive compounds give lettuce its healing and protective power. It's a rich source of omega-3 fatty acids and it offers skincare benefits.

The enzymes in lettuce provide the antibacterial properties that help to reduce the likelihood of bacterial infections of the skin, and the omega-3 can treat minor skin infections linked to acne.

Cabbage, another leafy green vegetable, is rich in vitamin B6 and folate!

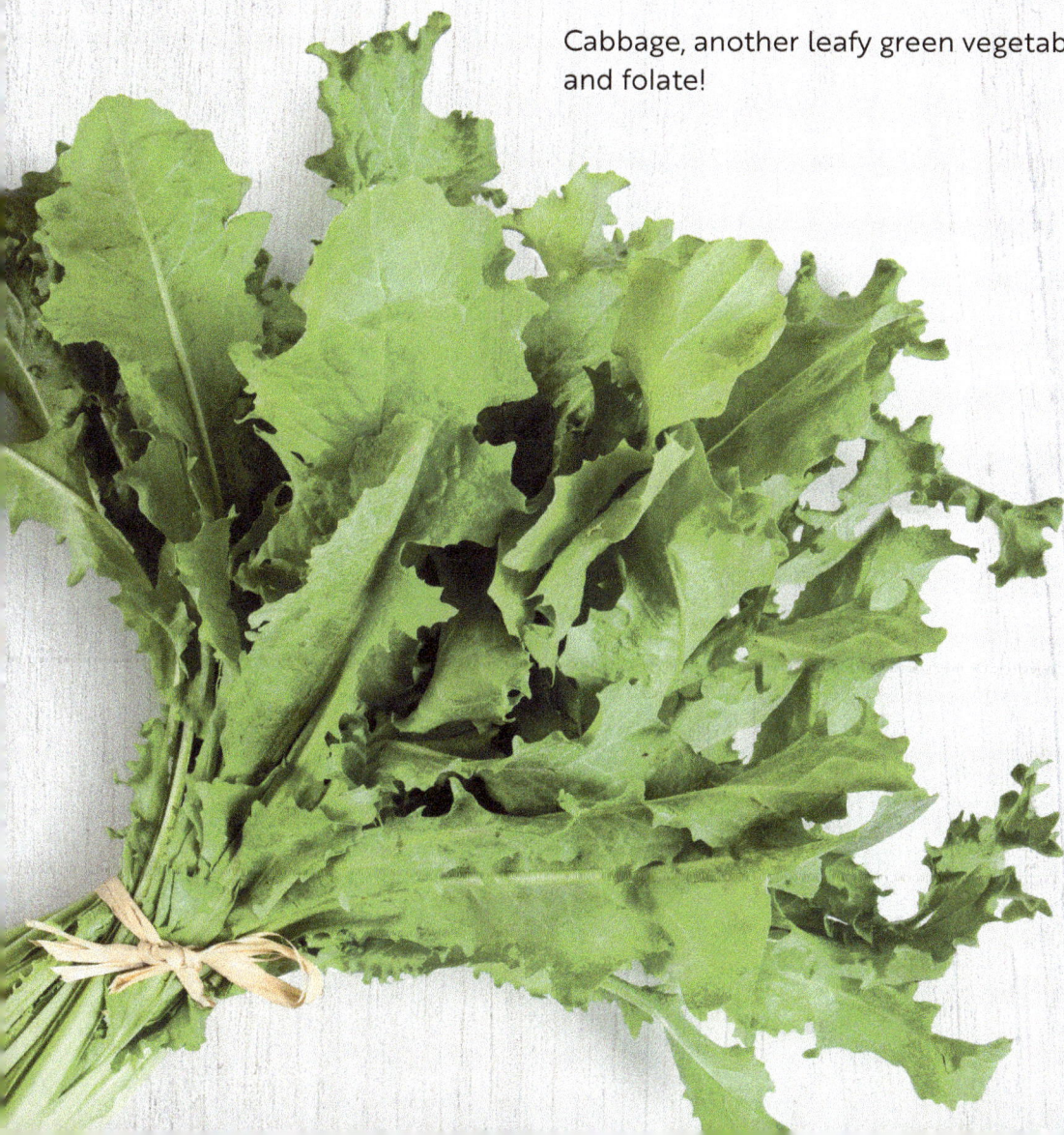

Parsley

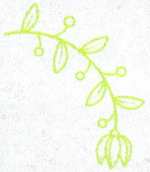

Strengthening the immune system is the first line of defence, which is undoubtedly needed, now more than ever! Sticking to your nutrition actually strengthens your immune system.

The plant kingdom

The plant kingdom (fruits, vegetables, herbs and spices) has lots of bright, vibrant colours, and many medicinal properties.

Do you suffer from digestive complaints? Parsley is a popular herb with many benefits, including high levels of vitamin C and vitamin K, and it helps strengthen the digestive system. It is also used as a diuretic, which can help prevent kidney stones.

The high levels of vitamin K found in parsley contribute to bone health and may reduce the risk of fractures. Evidently, this common herb's health benefits extend throughout the body.

I grew up in the produce industry, which meant that fresh fruits and vegetables were constantly available and taken for granted, until later in life when I studied natural medicine. I learned that nutrition is fundamental and the baseline of all sustained optimal health.

Lacking nutrition is an obstacle to cure if it is not acknowledged or addressed. Nutritional changes happen on the molecular level before they are seen on the physical plane, so don't give up; stay the course.

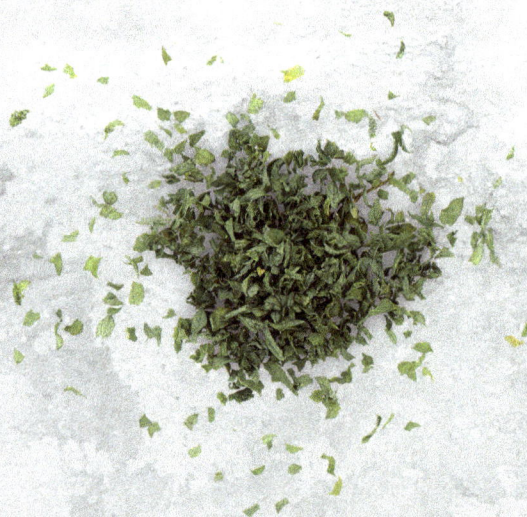

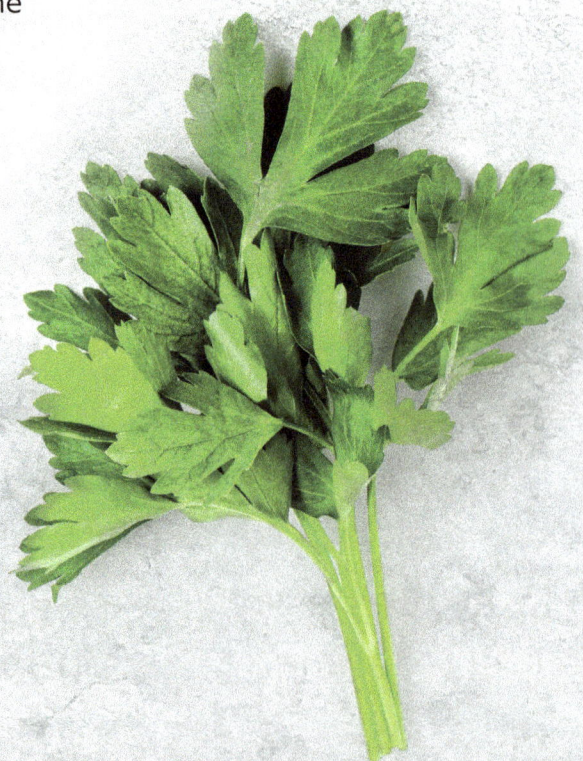

Anti-inflammatories

Some useful natural anti-inflammatories are turmeric, boswellia and glucosamine (which is used to repair joints and reduce pain). Cloves are also used to reduce inflammation and treat toothache.

Natural anti-inflammatory compounds inhibit inflammatory pathways, often with fewer side effects than some over-the-counter and prescription medications.

Cinnamon

One of nature's mighty antiseptics, cinnamon has strong antibacterial components. It is also known for its calming constituents and is thought to lower blood pressure.

Cinnamon is loaded with antioxidants, has anti-inflammatory properties, and may help protect against neurological disorders, such as Alzheimer's and Parkinson's. It's a versatile spice with a wide range of health benefits and medical uses.

Anise

Anise can be used to loosen mucus and clear the respiratory tract from congestion. Other uses of anise include relieving symptoms of bloating and digestive complaints. Anise is also said to promote speedy healing of acne scars and damaged skin, and it can minimise the appearance of fine lines and wrinkles.

Anise is rich in antioxidants and has anti-inflammatory, antibacterial, and antiviral properties. It is also a good source of minerals, including iron, calcium, and manganese.

Basil

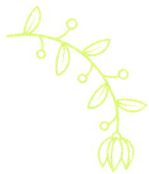

Basil is beneficial in the treatment of stress. A tea can be prepared with basil leaves, infused with sage leaves, and sweetened with honey. Basil has antispasmodic properties that make it useful for soothing an upset tummy and also help clear the nasal passages by stimulating the cilia in the nose.

Basil may provide a host of additional health benefits, including improved memory, reduced stress-related depression, and gut protection.

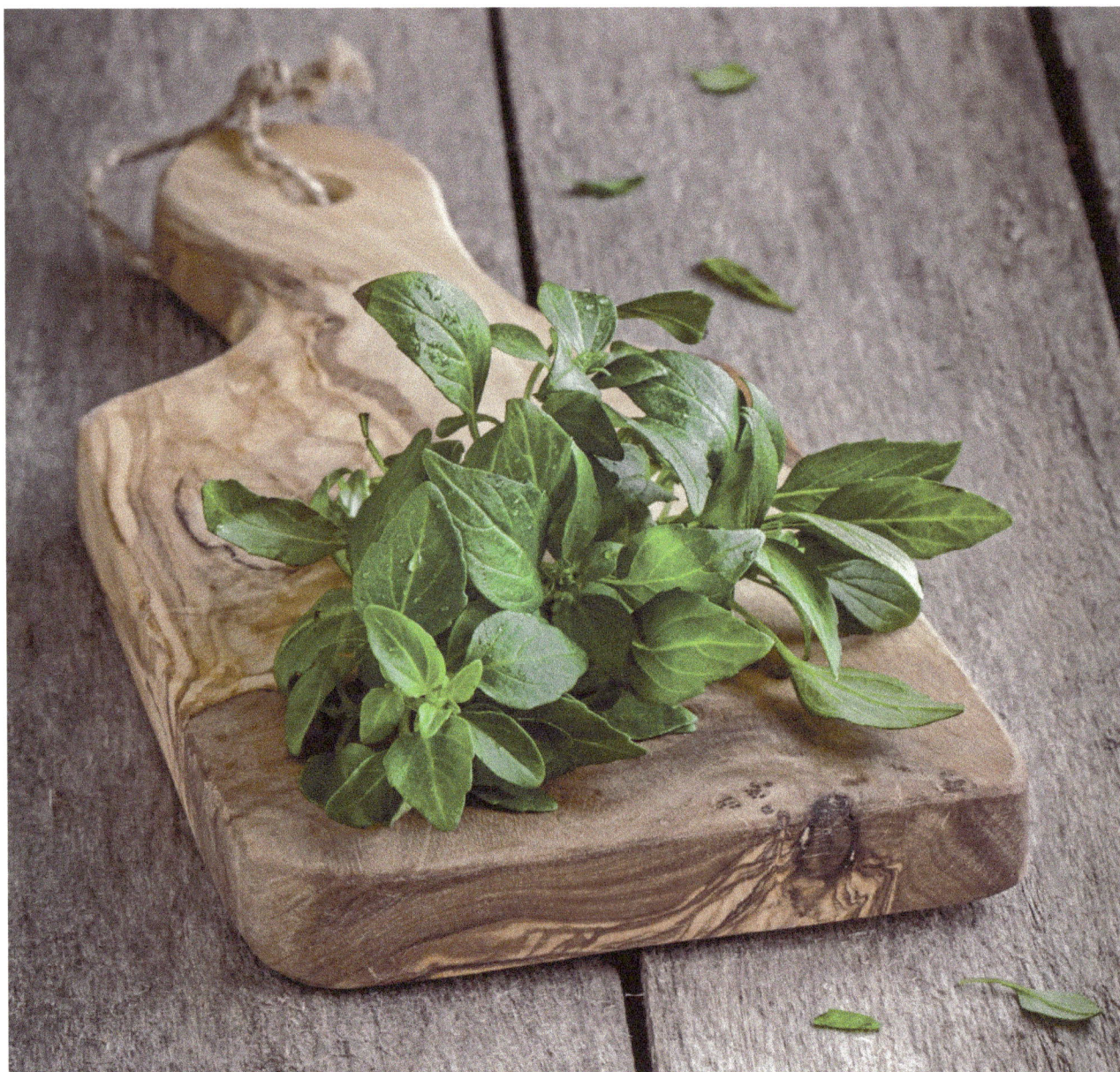

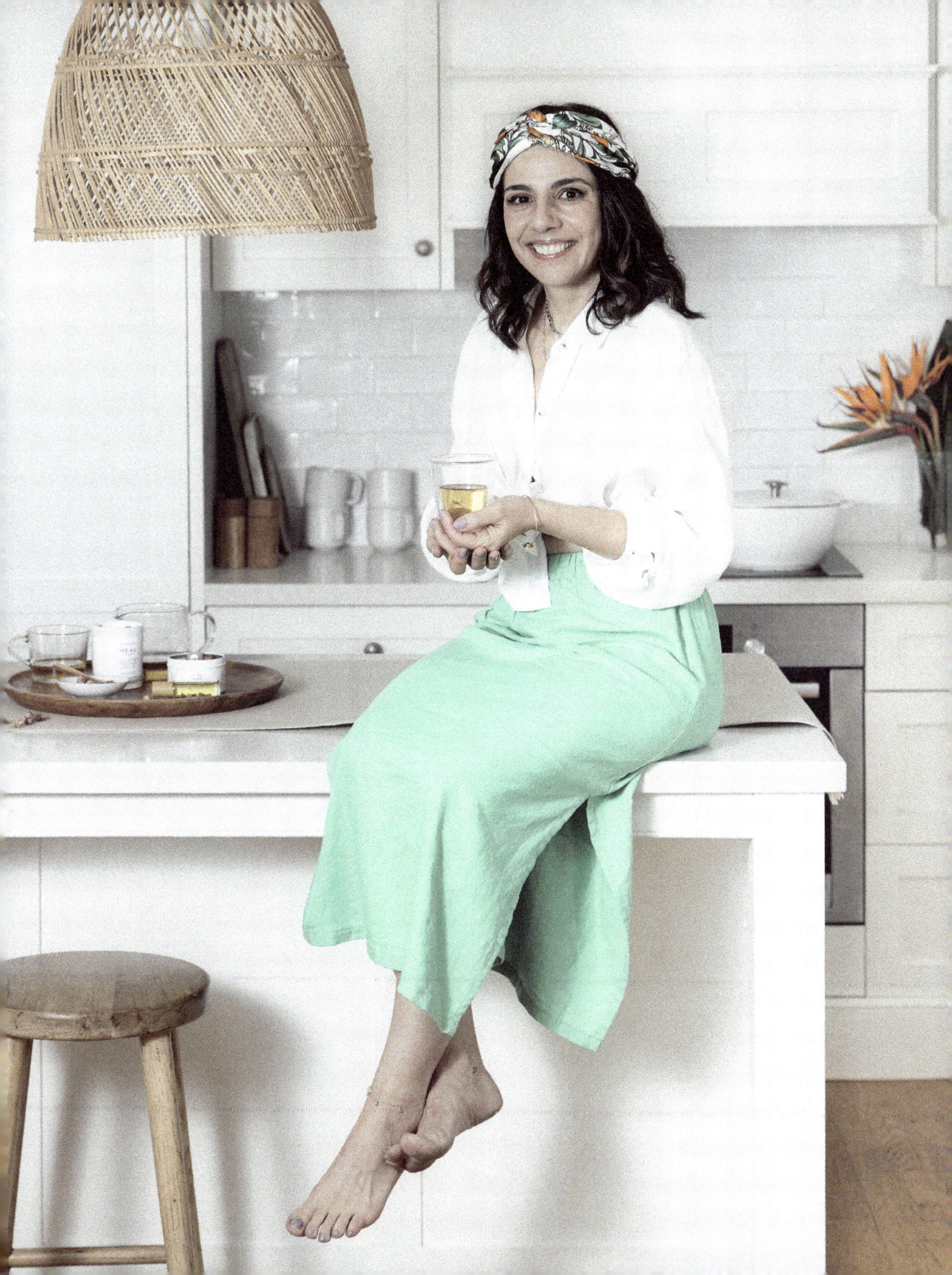

Nutritional minerals

Nutritional deficiency is an easily overlooked and common obstacle to cure. It is useful to become aware of the conditions that specific nutritional deficiencies can cause.

Homeopathic medicine has the capacity to enhance mineral absorption, but it is unlikely to be a substitute for frank deficiency. Don't overlook your nutrition.

Folic acid
Folate, or folic acid in its supplement form, contributes to the formation of DNA and RNA. During pregnancy, folate plays an important role in foetal development.

Folic acid deficiency is another obstacle to cure because our bodies don't make folate, so it needs to be obtained through our food or supplements. Deficiency has been known to cause or contribute to melasma.

HTMA
Hair Tissue Mineral Analysis is a non-intrusive health screening tool, showing reliable and clinical data on the Genova Diagnostics Nutrient and Toxic Elements Profile.

Causes of mineral imbalances can include diet, stress, medications, genetic factors, pollution and nutritional supplements.

Blood tests can give a good indication of the minerals being transported around the body, but they cannot accurately measure the minerals stored in tissue. This is particularly necessary when testing for toxic mineral exposure because the body removes them from the blood to protect us, and deposits them into tissues such as liver, bones, teeth, and hair.

The HTMA identifies toxic elements that have been sequestered out of blood and into tissue.

OligoScan

The OligoScan is another useful diagnostic tool for testing vitamin and element levels. It relies on a certain level of functional homeostasis and not on tissue excretion. OligoScan is noted as scanning for mineral density, precisely 4mm in depth of the peripheral tissues.

Once effective treatment begins via chelation and remineralisation, this mobilises toxic elements out of the deeper organ tissue and into the peripheral tissues, therefore, it is often recommended to have additional OligoScans after the initial scan to determine accurate levels as you move forward on your healing journey.

Copper

While zinc deficiency will predispose people to viruses, copper deficiency predisposes us to bacterial infections. Chronic bacterial infections can cause an endless cycle of infections that deplete copper stores even further.

Consuming foods that are high in copper, such as chocolate and Brazil nuts, can help with this deficiency.

However, copper excess is more common than deficiency and can be detected by a HTMA. Copper rises with oestrogen and can be retained in women using the OCP or IUD.

Excess copper also creates susceptibility to yeast infections, anxiety, depression, poor sleep, respiratory and food allergies.

Although not a common occurrence, copper deficiency creates a list of disorders that can be attributed to many chronic conditions. Therefore, its detection is most useful to both patient and practitioner. The list of issues includes immune response, reoccurring bacterial infection, musculoskeletal health, nervous system, and cardiovascular issues.

Overall, nutrition is incredibly important. The effects of unhealthy food consumption are not acute. Bad nutrition has slow, often silent and insidious effects; with long-term consequences which are then often treated symptomatically and labelled 'chronic' by conventional medicine.

This is not a
one size fits all
approach.

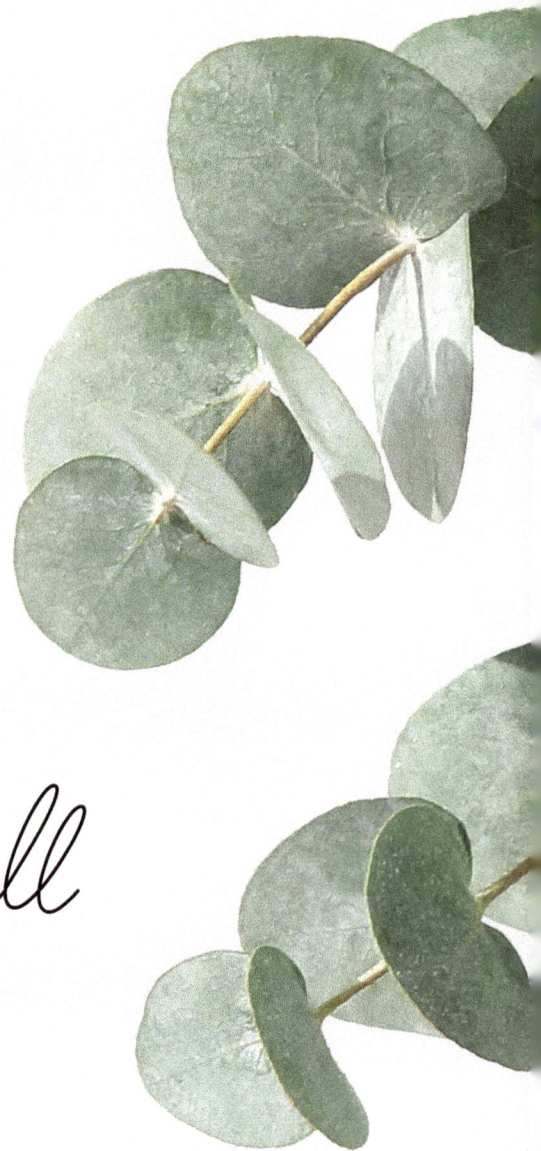

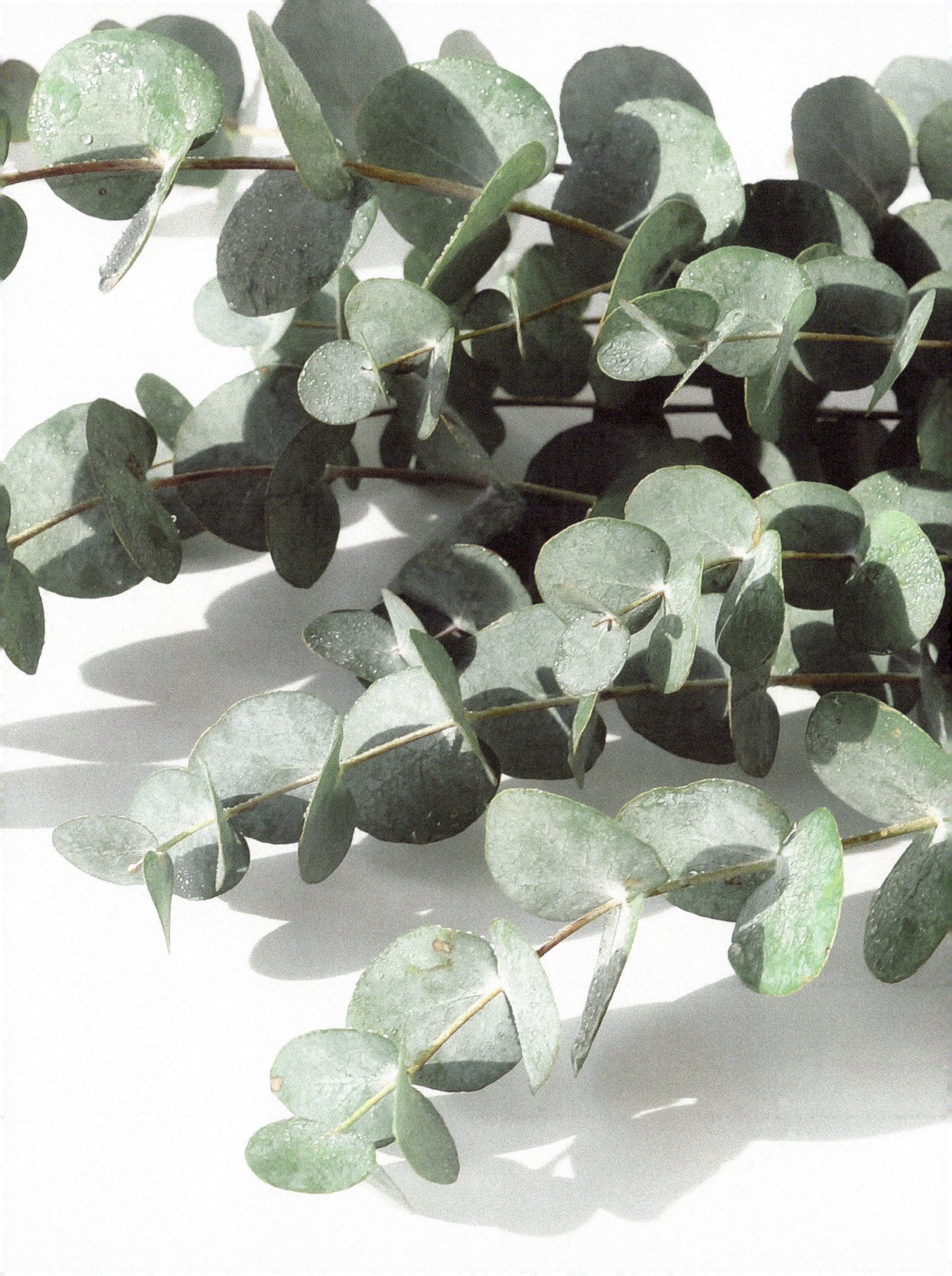

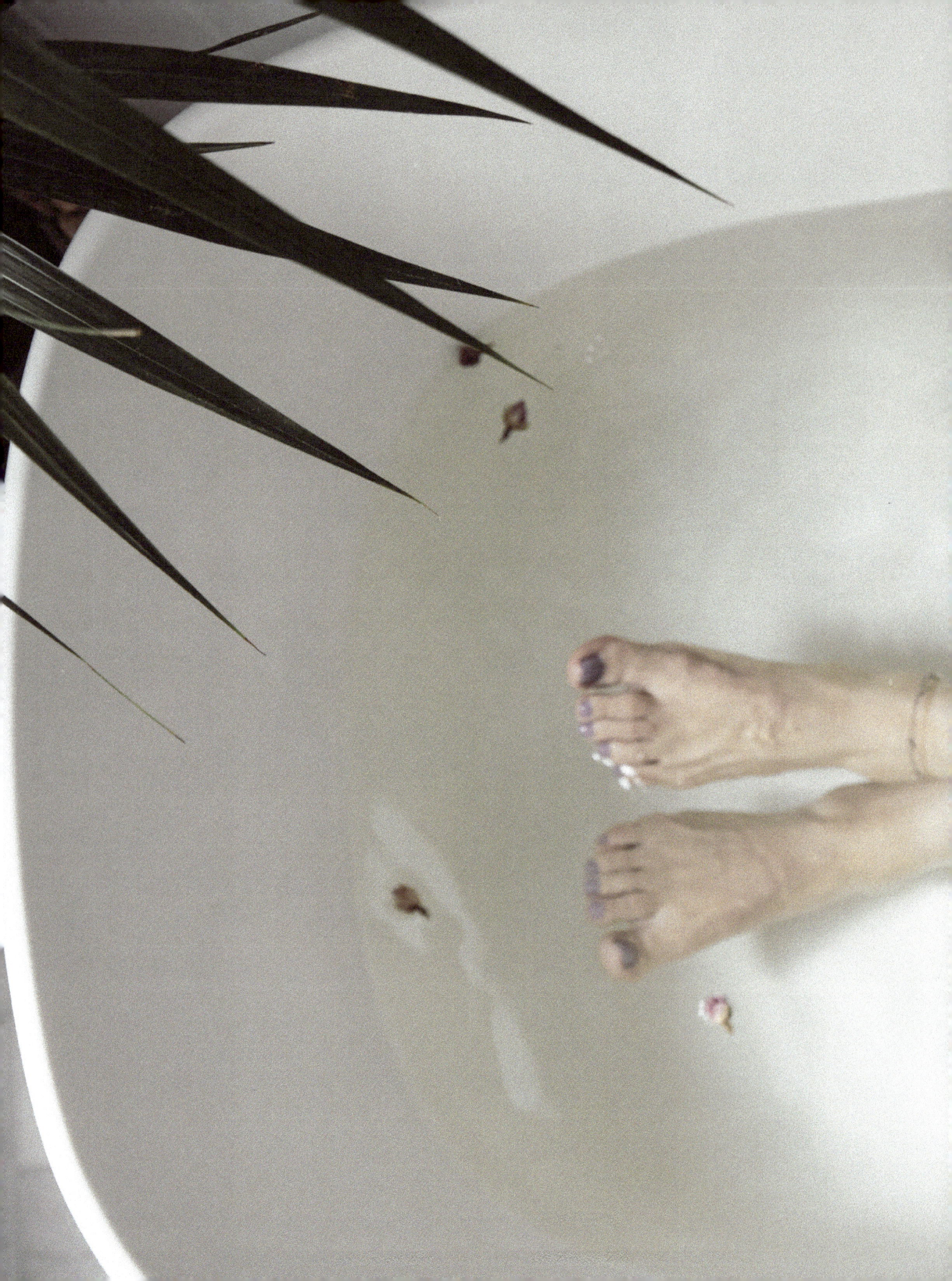

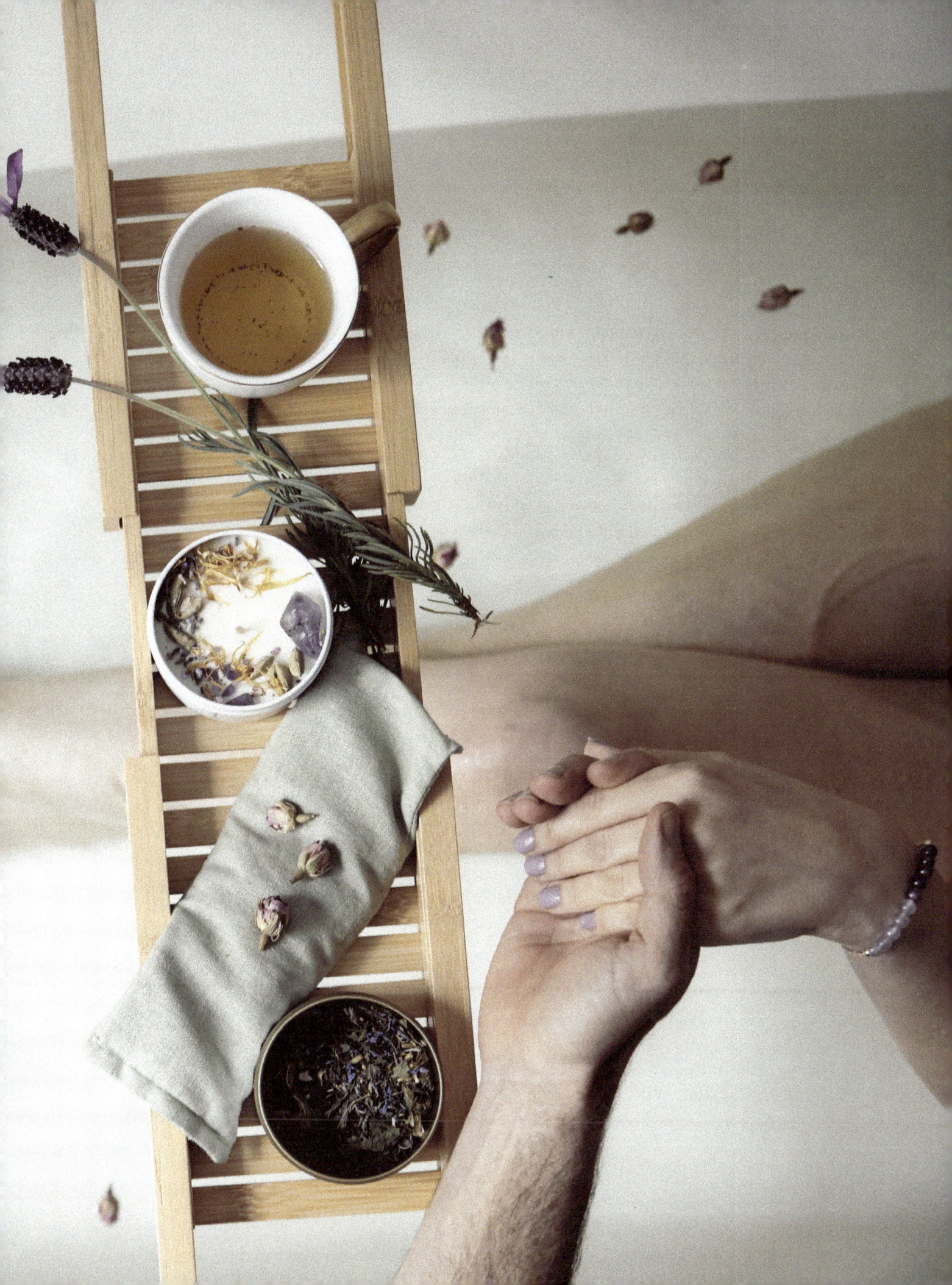

CONCLUSION

SHARE THIS BOOK

BONUS CONTENT

Homeopathy can help guide your body to heal itself.

I think our body stores emotion when there's too much to process or when something is too painful to look at in that moment. This is the dis-ease you are experiencing. The discord within.

Then when you do the work, you work on yourself, allowing the remedies to clear (sometimes years of) other stuck emotions that were also stored and in the way, and layer by layer you make your way through — clearing the path until you get to the one that was buried deep within, under all that was suppressing (protecting) it. It's been hiding behind your pain and it's coming up because you're ready to look at it now. Be with it and ask it what it needs.

Through the realisation and awareness of our patterns, gently being peeled back like layers of an onion, until you are there with your core truth — pure love.

YOU ARE THE MEDICINE
The life-giving healing light of the sun.
The rays of the moon.
The love in your heart.
Connect your bare feet to Mother Earth and tune in;
these are all avenues to deep power within you.

As you heal, you also heal the dynamics of your family and other relationships too.

Because, as your perception and behaviour is changing in a positive way, they respond differently to you and old patterns break. Your triggers are neutralised by the healing action of the remedies. This in itself is healing for everyone involved when all members of the family/relationship ecosystem have the same intention to heal.

The set fixed disturbed patterns around these relationship dynamics that cause you grief are dismantling. A pendulum shift has begun. Initially both pendulums were swinging in a specific pattern. Now one pendulum starts oscillating differently (in a healthier way), now the other has to follow with a new pattern. So, the entire relationship dynamic changes.

Thank you for giving me the opportunity to join you on your journey to heal. May it be blessed with divine guidance and love.

ACKNOWLEDGEMENTS

This goes out to all the Lionhearts.

My parents, Ben and Minnie, I am forever grateful for your continuous love and support ♥

My sisters, thank you for your encouragement over the years as I navigated my way through my own healing journey. You have always been my number one fans! Thank you ♥

My close friends and community who have stood by me, particularly in some of the most challenging times. These memories I will cherish forever ♡

A very big thank you to the team at Dean Publishing, particularly those I worked more closely with, for their kindness and professional expertise that helped me through this journey to become an author.

I would also like to thank the journey. The heartache, challenges, hurdles, closed doors, and people who made my life difficult; it is from these experiences that I have become the person I am today. These life lessons are the reason that I have journeyed where I have, experienced what I have, and acquired the knowledge and expertise that I have. The journey kept me searching, kept me hungry and determined, and eventually kept me motivated as it fuelled my fire. It is the reason for this book; without it, I would not have grown into the strong, capable woman that I am today, and I would not be able to help others.

I have written this book because the journey with all its glory and challenges has made me strong enough to HEAL.

ABOUT JOSEPHINE

Josephine Zappia, Adv.D.Hom.Med.
Sydney, Australia | Offering in-person and virtual services

Josephine is a practitioner of homeopathic medicine. With homeopathy's power to address the whole person, Josephine attracts patients who have not had success with conventional medicine, and who are spiritually aligned.

As a homeopath, Josephine connects with her patient's medical history and family medical history to determine the root cause and treatment of any dis-ease, addressing physical, mental, emotional, and spiritual aspects (as appropriate in each case). She also incorporates her wellness products that embrace herbal medicine and alchemical healing – these products include candles, oils and teas.

Josephine is passionate about healthcare and since experiencing her own healing journey, she discovered the importance of (and is keenly involved in) all other aspects of holistic health. This includes energy medicine - kinesiology, kundalini, vedic meditation, bodywork; a therapeutic practice relaxing the nervous system, shamanism, and sacred rebel spiritual healing.

Josephine is also trained in holistic counselling, but is not currently offering these services. She remains available for all other offerings.

WEBSITE   healbyjosephine.com

CONTACT   healbyjosephine.com/contact

INSTAGRAM   @healbyjosephine

LINKEDIN   www.linkedin.com/in/josephinezappia

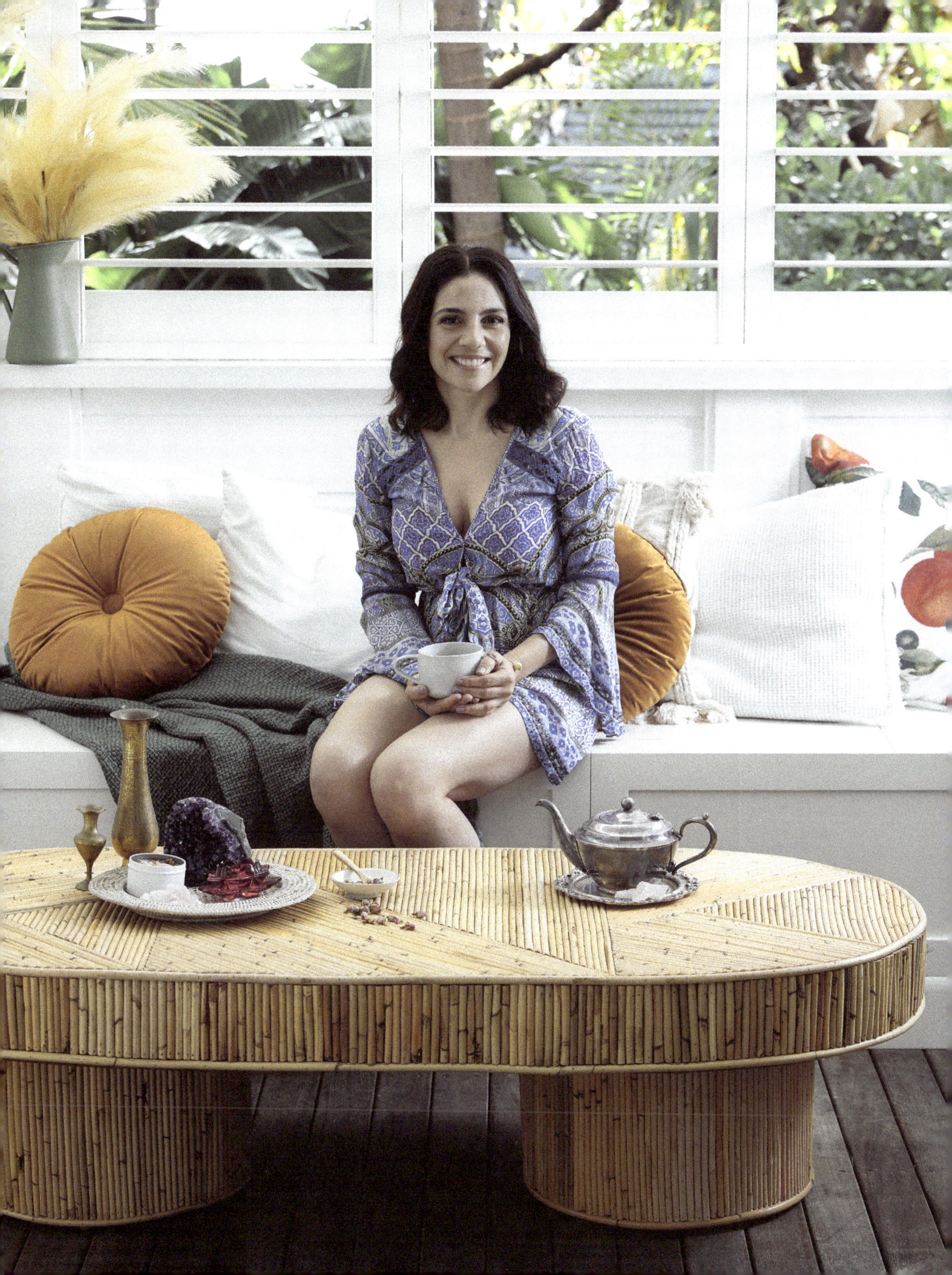

REFERENCES

Page 22: Crompton R. (2012). Homeopathy for common complaints during pregnancy and childbirth. *The practising midwife, 15*(8), S15–S18.Gregg D. Like cures like: homeopathy for labor and birth. Midwifery Today with International Midwife. 2010 (95):13-6, 64. PMID: 20949782.

Page 40: Anami Alchemia, [website] 'Sex Nectar: Herbal Tinctures - Scientific Studies', https://anami-alchemia.com/pages/studies, accessed August 14 2023.

Arentz, Susan et al. 'Herbal medicine for the management of polycystic ovary syndrome (PCOS) and associated oligo/amenorrhoea and hyperandrogenism; a review of the laboratory evidence for effects with corroborative clinical findings'. BMC complementary and alternative medicine vol. 14 511. 18 Dec. 2014, doi:10.1186/1472-6882-14-511

Jetmalani MH, Sabins PB, Gaitonde BB. 'A study on the pharmacology of various extracts of Shatavari-*Asparagus racemosus* (Willd)', *J Res Indian Med.* 1967;2:1–10.

Kashani L, Raisi F, Saroukhani S, et al. 'Saffron for treatment of fluoxetine-induced sexual dysfunction in women: Randomized double-blind placebo-controlled study'. *Hum Psychopharmacol Clin Exp.* 2012;28(1):54-60.

Lopresti, Adrian L, and Peter D Drummond. 'Saffron (Crocus sativus) for depression: a systematic review of clinical studies and examination of underlying antidepressant mechanisms of action.' Human psychopharmacology vol. 29,6 (2014): 517-27. doi:10.1002/hup.2434

Thakur, Mayank et al. 'A comparative study on aphrodisiac activity of some ayurvedic herbs in male albino rats.' Archives of sexual behavior vol. 38,6 (2009): 1009-15. doi:10.1007/s10508-008-9444-8

Sharma K, Bhatnagar M. *Asparagus racemosus* (Shatavari): 'A versatile female tonic', *Int J Pharm Biol Arch.* 2011;2(3):855–863.

Page 42-51: Kregiel D, Pawlikowska E, Antolak H. *Urtica* spp.: Ordinary plants with extraordinary properties. *Molecules.* 2018;23(7):1664. doi:10.3390/molecules23071664

Page 50: Ghasemzadeh Rahbardar, M & Hosseinzadeh, H 2020, 'Therapeutic effects of rosemary (*Rosmarinus officinalis* L.) and its active constituents on nervous system disorders', *Iranian Journal of Basic Medical Sciences*, vol 23, no 9, pp 1100–1112, https://doi.org/10.22038/ijbms.2020.45269.10541.

Page 51: Koulivand, PH, Khaleghi Ghadiri, M & Gorji, A 2013, 'Lavender and the nervous system', *Evidence-based Complementary and Alternative Medicine: eCAM*, vol 2013, p 681304, https://doi.org/10.1155/2013/681304.

Hamidpour, M, Hamidpour, R, Hamidpour, S & Shahlari, M 2014, 'Chemistry, pharmacology, and medicinal property of sage (salvia) to prevent and cure illnesses such as obesity, diabetes, depression, dementia, lupus, autism, heart disease, and cancer', *Journal of Traditional and Complementary Medicine*, vol 4, no 2, pp 82–88, https://doi.org/10.4103/2225-4110.130373.

Page 56: Pan, SY, Litscher, G, Gao, SH, Zhou, SF, Yu, ZL, Chen, HQ, Zhang, SF, Tang, MK, Sun, JN & Ko, KM 2014, 'Historical perspective of traditional indigenous medical practices: the current renaissance and conservation of herbal resources', *Evidence-based Complementary and Alternative Medicine: eCAM*, vol 2014, p 525340, https://doi.org/10.1155/2014/525340.

Robbins, Martin, 22 Nov, 2010, *The Guardian*, 'A challenge to homeopaths: how does one overdose?' https://www.theguardian.com/science/the-lay-scientist/2010/nov/21/1

Novella, S, Roy, R, Marcus, D, Bell IR, Davidovitch, N & Saine, A 2008, 'A debate: homeopathy – quackery or a key to the future of medicine?', *Journal of Alternative & Complementary Medicine*, vol 141, no 1, pp 9-15, https://doi.org/10.1089/acm.2007.0770.

Page 59: Turland, Jill, *Getting Back On Track: Using Megapotency Homeopathy*, 2021, Polaris Interstellar Digital Marketing.

Page 64: Oberbaum, M., Galoyan, N., Lerner-Geva, L., Singer, S. R., Grisaru, S., Shashar, D., & Samueloff, A. (2005). The effect of the homeopathic remedies Arnica montana and Bellis perennis on mild postpartum bleeding--a randomized, double-blind, placebo-controlled study--preliminary results. *Complementary therapies in medicine, 13*(2), 87–90. https://doi.org/10.1016/j.ctim.2005.03.006

Clarke, John Henry (1902) *A Dictionary of Practical Materia Medica, Volume 2*, Homœopathic Publishing Company.

Page 67: Timmerman, A & Jager, W 2012, 'Umbilical cord', *Homeopathic Links*, vol 25, no 4, pp 239-227, https://doi.org/10.1055/s-0032-1327857.

Page 68: Gibran, K 1923, *The Prophet*, Alfred A. Knopf, Inc, New York.

Page 69: Wang Y & Zhao S 2010, 'Vascular biology of the placenta', in DN Granger & JP Granger (eds), *Colloquium Series on Integrated Systems Physiology: From Molecule to Function to Disease*, Morgan & Claypool, San Rafael, CA, np, https://doi.org/10.4199/C00016ED1V01Y201008ISP009.

Page 70: Burns E 2014, 'More than clinical waste? Placenta rituals among Australian home-birthing women', *The Journal of Perinatal Education*, vol 23, no 1, pp 41–49, https://doi.org/10.1891/1058-1243.23.1.41.

Wang Y & Zhao S 2010, 'Vascular biology of the placenta', in DN Granger & JP Granger (eds), *Colloquium Series on Integrated Systems Physiology: From Molecule to Function to Disease*, Morgan & Claypool, San Rafael, CA, np, https://doi.org/10.4199/C00016ED1V01Y201008ISP009.

The Welsh School of Homeopathy, 'Placenta Humanum' [website 'Provings'] https://welshschoolofhomeopathy.org.uk/provings/Placenta.pdf

Page 72: Martin, CR, Ling, PR & Blackburn, GL 2016, 'Review of infant feeding: Key features of breastmilk and infant formula', *Nutrients*, vol 8, no 5, p 279, https://doi.org/10.3390/nu8050279.

Page 73: Razlog, R, Pellow, J, Patel, R, Caminsky, M & Van Heerden, HJ 2016, 'Case studies on the homeopathic treatment of binge eating in adult males', *Health SA Gesondheid*, vol 21, pp 294-302, https://doi.org/10.1016/j.hsag.2016.06.006.

Page 77: Dinsmoor, MJ, Viloria, R, Lief, L & Elder, S 2005, 'Use of intrapartum antibiotics and the incidence of postnatal maternal and neonatal yeast infections', *Obstetrics and Gynecology*, vol 106, no 1, pp 19–22, https://doi.org/10.1097/01.AOG.0000164049.12159.bd.

Page 84: Hahnemann, S 2010, *Organon of Medicine*, 5th and 6th edn, RE Dudgeon & W Boericke (trans), B. Jain Publishers, New Delhi.

Page 86: Foubister's pamphlet; Foubister's Tutorials; O.A. Julian; Sankaran; Boericke; Coulter, Vol.2

Page 98-99: Sankaran, Rajan, *The Other Song: Discovering Your Parallel Self*, 2008, Homoeopathic Medical Publishers.

Sankaran, Rajan, HPathy.com. March 18, 2017, 'Understanding The Kingdom Classification: Introduction to the Mineral, Plant and Animal Kingdoms' [website] https://hpathy.com/materia-medica/understanding-kingdom-classification-introduction-mineral-plant-animal-kingdoms/

Page 100: Welling, LLM, 2013, 'Psychobehavioral effects of hormonal contraceptive use', *Evolutionary Psychology*, vol 11, no 3, pp 718-742, https://doi.org/10.1177/147470491301300110.

Berg, G, Kohlmeier, L & Brenner, H 1998, 'Effect of oral contraceptive progestins on serum copper concentration', *European Journal of Clinical Nutrition*, vol 52, no 10, pp 711–715, https://doi.org/10.1038/sj.ejcn.1600631.

Page 107: quote is from William H. Burt, MD and is a summary of his findings in clinical practice

Page 108: Welte, U 2016, *Colours in Homeopathy: Colour Repertory with Instructions*, Narayana Publishers, Kandern, Germany.

Page 112-113: Hahnemann, S 2010, *Organon of Medicine*, 5th and 6th edn, RE Dudgeon & W Boericke (trans), B. Jain Publishers, New Delhi.

McKay, LI & Cidlowski, JA 2003, 'Physiologic and pharmacologic effects of corticosteroids', in DW Kufe, RE Pollock & RR Weichselbaum (eds), *Holland-Frei Cancer Medicine*, 6th edn, BC Decker, Ontario.

Rozencwajg, Joe Dr 2015, *Elementary Nutrition for Homeopaths*, Lulu Publishing.

Zhou, SS, Li, D, Zhou, YM & Cao, JM 2012, 'The skin function: a factor of anti-metabolic syndrome', *Diabetology & Metabolic Syndrome*, vol 4, no 1, p 15, https://doi.org/10.1186/1758-5996-4-15.

Page 114-115: Gamble, Jon, *Mastering Homeopathy 3 - Obstacles to Cure: Toxicity, Deficiency and Infection* 2010, Karuna Publishing.

Page 115: Lei, L, Su, J, Chen, J, Chen, W, Chen, X & Peng, C 2019, 'Abnormal serum copper and zinc levels in patients with psoriasis: A meta-analysis', *Indian Journal of Dermatology*, vol 64, no 3, pp 224–230, https://doi.org/10.4103/ijd.IJD_475_18.

Jameson, S 1976, 'Zinc deficiency in malabsorption states: a cause of infertility?', *Acta Medica Scandinavica. Supplementum*, vol 593, pp 38–49, https://doi.org/10.1111/j.0954-6820.1976.tb12825.x.

Petrilli, MA, Kranz, TM, Kleinhaus, K, Joe, P, Getz, M, Johnson, P, Chao, MV & Malaspina, D 2017, 'The emerging role for zinc in depression and psychosis', *Frontiers in Pharmacology*, vol 8, p 414, https://doi.org/10.3389/fphar.2017.00414.

REFERENCES

Pages 116-132: McCosker, Kim, Bermingham, Rachael, Chopra Deepak, *4 Ingredients: Fast, Fresh and Healthy*, 2010, Hay House.

Page 117: Veisi, Parisa & Zarezade, Meysam & Rostamkhani, Helya & Ghoreishi, Zohreh. (2022). Renoprotective effects of the ginger (Zingiber officinale) on Diabetic kidney disease, current knowledge and future direction: a systematic review of animal studies. *BMC Complementary Medicine and Therapies*. 22. 10.1186/s12906-022-03768-x.

Page 120: Ma, ZF & Lee, YY 2016, 'Virgin coconut oil and its cardiovascular health benefits', *Natural Product Communications*, vol 11, no 8, pp 1151-1152, https://doi.org/10.1177/1934578X1601100829.

Peedikayil, FC, Remy, V, John, S, Chandru, TP, Sreenivasan, P & Bijapur, GA 2016, 'Comparison of antibacterial efficacy of coconut oil and chlorhexidine on *Streptococcus mutans*: An *in vivo* study', *Journal of International Society of Preventive & Community Dentistry*, vol 6, no 5, pp 447–452, https://doi.org/10.4103/2231-0762.192934.

Page 122-123: Bonaz, B, Bazin, T & Pellissier, S 2018, 'The vagus nerve at the interface of the microbiota-gut-brain axis', *Frontiers in Neuroscience*, vol 12, p 49, https://doi.org/10.3389/fnins.2018.00049

Kharrazian, Datis, 2017, 'Unwinding Leaky Gut' - Kharrazian Resource Centre, [online], https://drknews.com/about-dr-datis-kharrazian/

Leyva-López, N, Gutiérrez-Grijalva, EP, Vazquez-Olivo, G & Heredia, JB 2017, 'Essential oils of oregano: Biological activity beyond their antimicrobial properties', *Molecules (Basel, Switzerland)*, vol 22, no 6, p 989, https://doi.org/10.3390/molecules22060989.

Barbaro, B, Toietta, G, Maggio, R, Arciello, M, Tarocchi, M, Galli, A & Balsano, C 2014, 'Effects of the olive-derived polyphenol oleuropein on human health', *International Journal of Molecular Sciences*, vol 15, no 10, pp 18508–18524, https://doi.org/10.3390/ijms151018508.

Page 128: Chan JY, Yuen AC, Chan RY & Chan SW 2013, 'A review of the cardiovascular benefits and antioxidant properties of allicin', *Phytotherapy Research*, vol 27, pp 637–646.

Page 131: Khasnavis, S., & Pahan, K. (2014). Cinnamon treatment upregulates neuroprotective proteins Parkin and DJ-1 and protects dopaminergic neurons in a mouse model of Parkinson's disease. *Journal of neuroimmune pharmacology : the official journal of the Society on NeuroImmune Pharmacology*, 9(4), 569–581. https://doi.org/10.1007/s11481-014-9552-2

Page 134: Greenberg, JA, Bell, SJ, Guan, Y & Yu, YH 2011, 'Folic acid supplementation and pregnancy: more than just neural tube defect prevention', *Reviews in Obstetrics & Gynecology*, vol 4, no 2, pp 52–59.

Page 135: Gamble, Jon, *Mastering Homeopathy 3 - Obstacles to Cure: Toxicity, Deficiency and Infection* 2010, Karuna Publishing.

Gamble, Jon, *Mastering Chronic Disease: Toxicity, Deficiency and Infection,* 2022, Karuna Publishing.

Luxometrix-ipc.eu Société Anonyme 2013, *Oligoscan*, webpage, http://www.oligoscan.fr/

National Research Council (US) Committee on Copper in Drinking Water 2000, 'Health Effects of Excess Copper', in *Copper in Drinking Water*, National Academies Press, Washington DC, https://www.ncbi.nlm.nih.gov/books/NBK225400/.

JOURNAL